fat-burner workout

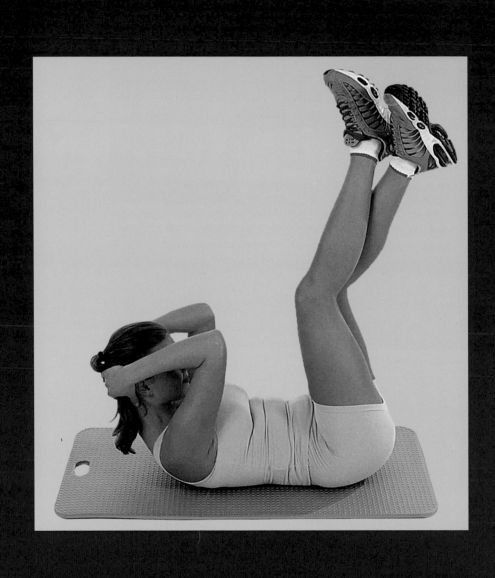

fat–burner workout

Chrissie Gallagher-Mundy

BB **Bounty**
BOOKS

First published in Great Britain in 2003 by Hamlyn, a division
of Octopus Publishing Group Ltd

Copyright © 2003 Octopus Publishing Group Ltd

This edition published in 2004 by Bounty Books, a division of
Octopus Publishing Group Ltd
2–4 Heron Quays, London E14 4JP
Reprinted 2005

ISBN   0 7537 1038 2

ISBN13   9780753710388

A catalogue record for this book is available from the British
Library.

Printed and bound in China

Note
Whilst the advice and information in this book is believed to
be accurate, neither the author nor the publisher will be
responsible for any injury, losses, damages, actions,
proceedings, claims, demands, expenses and costs (including
legal costs or expenses) incurred or in any way arising out of
following the exercises in this book.

Contents

Introduction

We all want to have good-looking bodies, but what exactly is a good body? Defined muscles and a relatively low level of body fat make up the shape that most men and women aspire to. But there is some confusion as to how to build the best muscle tone, and many people struggle with the problem of keeping their body fat (and therefore their weight) down.

This book aims to give you the best available advice on how to become strong and lean. In addition to providing information on healthy eating and dieting, it provides you with practical ways of working out and exercising regularly, which are the keys to a slim and fit body. This will not only give you the shape that looks good but also a strong body frame in the best condition for a long, healthy life. The book encourages you to exercise and eat (preferably little and often) regularly – every day if possible. With regular exercise and food input your body learns to be an efficient fat-burner and the metabolism stays raised.

If you want to get the best out of your body, then this is the book for you. You must, however, be realistic about what you can achieve with what you have to work with.

A realistic look at yourself

When starting on a body fat reduction programme it is very important to be realistic. If you want to be taller, have longer legs or larger breasts – this book cannot help you. If, however, you want to tone up your arms and legs and reduce the amount of excess fat you are carrying around your body – then read on!

Don't be fooled into thinking there are too many short cuts, because there usually aren't. These things are dictated by birth: height and underlying build are predetermined and we are all at the mercy of what we inherit. What you can do is make the best of what you've got. It is amazing what a change lessening the body fat can make. By toning, losing body fat and shaping different areas you can make yourself appear taller, slimmer and stronger than your original genes may have allowed for.

As you learn to slot more activity into your daily life, exercise will become as much a natural part of your routine as eating.

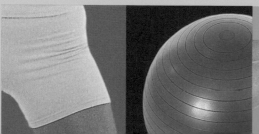
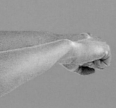
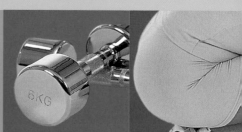

It's all in the genes

▶ Height, length of limbs and skin tone are all dictated by genetics and heredity. They are the characteristics we cannot change.

▶ Basic musculature and proportion of body fat is also passed down to us in our genes, as are our metabolism and propensity to activity. These, however, are things we do have some control over.

What's the book about?

The first three chapters of this book provide an understanding of fat and what to do to control it. Chapters 1 and 2 look at exactly what fat is, how to measure it and the dangers of being over-fat, before studying the principles of losing body fat through exercise – both aerobic and anaerobic. We discuss the intensity of the workout required and the role of the body's metabolism in losing body fat, as well as listing the general components of a fat-burning fitness programme. Chapter 3 introduces the latest advice on how to eat sensibly, especially when exercising.

Chapter 4 is the focus of this book – a full 30-day fitness programme with step-by-step exercises that will guide you through a month of solid fat-burning training. The programme assumes you do not have limitless time to exercise – most of us have to fit our exercise regime around 101 other things – so it encourages you to burn as many calories as you can in the shortest time possible. Day 1 starts from a point of relative un-fitness and the exercises vary from day to day, but each one includes an aerobic or anaerobic element for pure calorie burning and a 'Muscle Strengthener' for toning. For the best results, follow the programme over 30 consecutive days, but you could follow it every other day, if you preferred.

The final chapter suggests ways of fitting a higher level of activity into your everyday life – exercising while at work, on holiday, and even in front of the television.

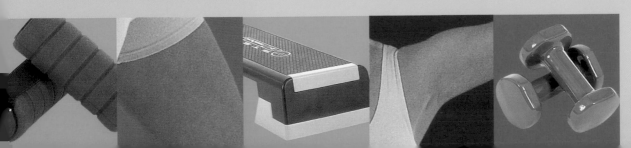

7

8

1 Facts about fat

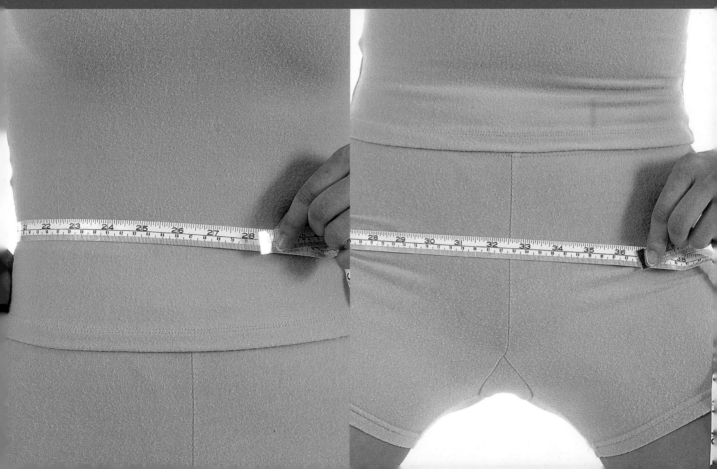

Fat or thin?

'Fat' is one of the buzzwords of modern times. It is a word that is used and overused by advertisers and the media alike to refer to body shapes and to sell body-shaping products. When we use the words 'fat' and 'thin' to describe someone's physique, it is 'thin' we are always hoping for. 'Fat' has become a derogatory term and there is no end of hype over who is fat, what is fat, whether one should be fat and if so, to what degree.

Through the ages

This wasn't always the case. Historically, fat was, and indeed in certain other cultures, still is, acceptable and even desirable. If you look at the work of the painter Rubens and his contemporaries in the 17th century you will see paintings of buxom young women with rippling flesh, who were considered beautiful at that time. In some African cultures, to be fat is to be well fed, which implies wealth and health.

At other times in history fashion has decreed that women should look thinner in some places and fatter in others, for instance the tiny waists created by corsets, or the full backsides that were emphasized by the skirts and bustles worn in the late 19th century. In the 1960s, on the other hand, it suddenly became the height of fashion to be stick thin with no curves or roundness at all.

Part of the problem with fashion nowadays is that we all show a lot more of our actual bodies. Any modern fashion therefore has to be wrought on the body rather than be achieved by the careful use of clothes. So far, this preference for a slim shape has prevailed and has now been given support by scientists who are interested in our health rather than fashion.

Medical thinking

As science has advanced and medical understanding improved, the message now is that for a person to remain healthy a certain optimum body weight needs to be maintained. While in some cultures, fat people may be seen as healthy, the growing evidence is that very fat people are prone to suffer many more health problems. In the western world, life expectancy is lengthening, and with this fact comes the need

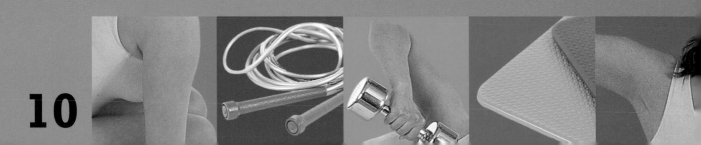

to keep our bodies working well into old age so that we do not spend the last ten years of our lives with our minds racing but our bodies immobile!

Modern lifestyles

It is ironic that while fashion and science are putting pressure on both men and women to be slim and slimmer, we have reached an age where the necessity to move is ever decreasing and the abundance of over-fattening foods is increasing every day. While cavemen and women kept naturally fit and agile by having to run off and hunt for their food, today's western lifestyle means we have everything at the touch of a button. We jump in a car to go to the corner shop. We don't get up to change the television channel because we have a remote control and if we want to go up flights of stairs or on walks there are escalators and moving walkways so that we need hardly move at all!

In addition to this, food is more plentiful and more tempting than ever before. Wherever we go we are bombarded with all kinds of new and enticing food choices, some of which are not necessarily the best for our bodies.

These are the main reasons why many people struggle with the issue of fat and keeping their weight down today. As we do less and eat more, gaining weight has become something that our modern race has to struggle against, as much as cavemen needed to struggle against starvation.

Benefits of being a healthy weight

▶ You avoid putting extra pressure on the spinal column and joints, which can lead to injuries and back problems.

▶ You will move more easily, with more dynamism and have more zest for life.

▶ Joints not restricted by extra flesh will optimize your flexibility.

▶ You reduce your risk of developing diabetes, stroke, high cholesterol and high blood pressure.

▶ You will look and feel good.

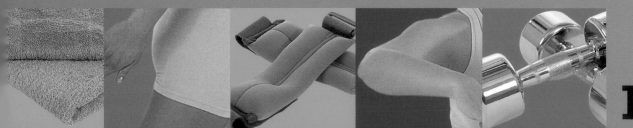

Fat facts

Don't be fooled into thinking that all body fat is bad. It is only in excess that it is bad. The body needs a skeletal frame with muscles attached via tendons and ligaments to produce movement. Some fat is also essential, to cushion internal organs, provide warmth and allow us to store energy for later use.

When we are born the body is made up of approximately 12 per cent fat. This can increase to 30 per cent by the age of six months. As the baby grows into an active toddler, the body fat naturally decreases so the percentage may reduce to around 18 per cent.

By young adulthood the body fat percentage should probably be around 20–25 per cent for women and 13–18 per cent for men. Women carry more fat than men to facilitate childbearing, and around puberty they tend to lay down fat around their breasts, hips, thighs and buttocks. At this time men tend to gain in muscle.

This ratio of body fat to lean muscle mass should ideally be maintained for the rest of one's adult life.

Becoming fat

The build-up of body fat that is not needed usually occurs in adulthood, when we tend to focus so much more on food. We look forward to it, may have to plan and prepare it, and stop working for it. Many of our psychological breaks come from someone saying: 'Time for tea!'

As we take in excess food, we take in more energy (calories) than we need. The excess gets stored in the body in fat cells in the adipose tissue, just beneath the skin. This excess is stored until such time as there may be starvation or a need for a huge expenditure of energy. It is both a problem and a blessing of modern life that these circumstances rarely occur in the western world. Therefore while our lives are less stressed by life-threatening 'fight or flight' situations and we don't go through days of starvation, the downside is that our bodies become neglected and overfed, which begins to slow us down.

As we retain excess energy as body fat we expand the cells that hold the fat. When they get full,

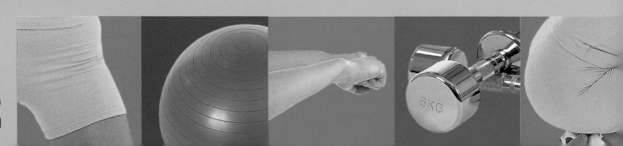

the vicious fat circle

less activity undertaken

more fat stored

less energy used

the cells divide to form new fat cells ready to be filled. These cells, once created, never go away. As the fat cells become full, the sugar, fat and protein can spill over into the bloodstream, causing the body to create yet more fat cells.

Vicious circle

With more cells full of fat, we grow heavier, and general activity becomes more of an effort. So we sit on the sofa more and walk less because it makes our muscles ache and our bodies tire. The less activity we do, the less energy is used up and the more that is stored in the fat cells. As we increase in size, we can't bend and twist so well, the spine takes more weight and is more stressed. Because of the current trend for slim body shapes we may also become embarrassed or self-conscious at attempting any form of exercise and consequently we become more sedentary and fatter still!

Fat storage

Different people tend to store fat in different parts of the body. Genetics and other hereditary factors dictate this (see pages 14–15). Men tend to store their fat around the middle of the body, giving rise to the 'beer gut' look. It is from here that fat is more readily released into the bloodstream, and this can lead to an increased risk of heart attacks and strokes. In women, the tendency has been for the fat to be stored in the lower regions – giving rise to the pear-shaped figure. This has its advantages as fat is less metabolically active here.

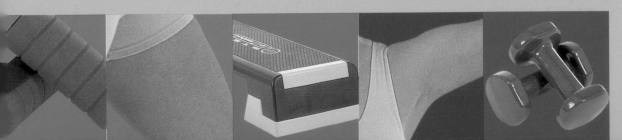

Defining your body type

Many things affect where and how your body stores fat. One of them may be the type of body you have inherited. Dr William H. Sheldon, working in the 1940s, first introduced the notion of somatotypes, which puts body types into three categories.

These three types are called ectomorph, mesomorph and endomorph. While they are not scientifically defined, they give you an idea of what kind of body you have to work with. This should not be taken too seriously; what it can help you with, however, is defining your goals at the beginning of a programme.

When you have a clear idea of what body type you are working with (see box, right), you will have a better idea of what you can achieve. This way you won't be working for inappropriate goals that set you up for failure – but goals that suit your frame and thus show faster results.

Ectomorph

This body type tends to be thinner and more fragile with a delicate or lightly muscled frame. People of this type tend to be taller and can be stoop shouldered. Muscle growth in this type takes longer.

If this is your type then you will need to work harder at building muscle and working on postural alignment. When you use the 30-day programme in Chapter 4 you can emphasize these aspects of the suggested training.

Mesomorph

This body type tends to be athletic-looking with a harder, muscular appearance. Some mesomorph women can be rectangular or hourglass-shaped with a thicker skin and upright posture. People of this type grow muscle quickly and can usually lose (or gain) weight easily, too.

If this is your type, toning up may happen quickly and if you do the 30-day programme, losing body fat should happen, too. Emphasize the cardiovascular (CV) side of your training to keep your heart and CV system in top shape.

Endomorph

This body type tends towards a soft body that can be flabby. Muscles tend to be less developed and the shape rounded. It is usually harder for these types to lose weight but they can gain muscle relatively easily.

If this is your type then you need to work hard on muscle-building, which will help with fat loss. You need to work consistently to build the muscle – it takes six to eight weeks to build new muscle – which will define your shape and help use up calories.

Ectomorph, mesomorph or endomorph?

Assess your bone structure by wrapping your hand around your wrist and seeing where the thumb and middle finger reach. If they don't touch, you are probably a large frame; if they just touch you are a medium frame; if they overlap you are a small frame.

Now assess your body shape by looking in the mirror. Wearing a thin T-shirt and leggings, stand squarely in front of the glass and observe.

Ask yourself the following questions:

1 Is your bone structure and figure generally:
- **A** large
- **B** medium
- **C** small to frail?

2 Think about when you were a child and also in the last ten years. Has your body always tended towards:
- **A** carrying too much fat
- **B** being lean and muscular
- **C** being skinny or slight?

3 Do you:
- **A** gain weight easily and find it harder to lose
- **B** usually stay about the same weight
- **C** have trouble gaining weight or losing it easily?

What do the answers mean?

If you answered mainly **A**, the chances are you are an **endomorph**.

If you answered mainly **B**, the chances are you are a **mesomorph**.

If you answered mainly **C**, the chances are you are an **ectomorph**.

If your answers were **divided** then your body shape will be a **combination** of types.

The dangers of being fat

While we should not be slaves to the extreme fashion for thinness, and should be aware that many overweight people live perfectly normal lives, it is important to be as healthy as possible in order to maintain the quality and length of our lives.

We tend not to value our health until we temporarily lose it. It is something we take for granted, yet it takes only a bad hangover to remind you what bad health is like and to make you swear you will never drink again! In the same way, we are all much more aware nowadays of the kinds of foods that are beneficial to the body and the importance of exercise. Yet we find it hard to put this into practice.

Healthwise, there are some pretty compelling arguments for maintaining a regular programme of exercise and a healthy diet.

Diabetes

Diabetes is a disease where the body is unable to maintain normal blood sugar (glucose) levels naturally. Sufferers may have too little insulin in their blood (Type 1 or insulin dependent diabetes) or too much (Type 2 or non insulin dependent diabetes). This causes an overproduction of blood glucose, which in turn acts on many organs to produce the various symptoms of diabetes.

Type 1 diabetics (five to ten per cent of diabetics) need regular injections to boost their insulin levels. Type 2, or adult-onset, diabetes (90 per cent of all sufferers) is where the body becomes insulin resistant.

Not only do diabetics have to manage their own blood sugar levels, but they are at increased risk from many health problems such as kidney failure, nerve disorder, eye problems and heart disease. The risk of becoming diabetic is greatly increased if you are over-fat as insulin resistance is linked to obesity.

For the diabetic, keeping body fat under control and exercising regularly is paramount. For the non-insulin dependent diabetic, lifestyle changes involving proper diet and exercise control play an important role in management of the disease.

While exercise may not prevent diabetes or its attendant problems, it can improve the health of the heart and keep the patient de-stressed while they manage the disease.

Impaired glucose tolerance (IGT)

IGT is where the blood glucose levels are higher than normal but not yet diabetic. The risk of people becoming diabetic rises as patients become increasingly sedentary and over-fat.

High blood pressure

The two numbers in a blood pressure reading measure the maximum output pressure of the heart and the pressure when the heart is at rest. Numbers that are too high indicate that the heart is having to work too hard because of restrictions or a loss of elasticity in the coronary arteries.

High blood pressure can make the heart fail through overwork and causes kidney failure. While there are many reasons for high blood pressure, being over-fat, under-fit and stressed are all risk factors.

When you exercise you cut down on all these risks. Exercise builds muscle, which requires additional calories to maintain it, and increases the metabolism. Aerobic exercise (see page 26) uses stored fat to keep up energy levels and helps with fat control. Exercise will leave you feeling refreshed and less stressed.

Some people who suffer from high blood pressure are actually able to cut down on their blood pressure medications thanks to regular exercise and diet management.

Heart disease

Heart disease is any condition that causes your heart to malfunction. Most commonly it refers to

Healthy living

Remember that for all diseases there are general risks such as age and genetics. Yet these risks are definitely worsened by:

▶ Smoking

▶ A high-fat diet

▶ Being overweight and over-fat

coronary artery disease. This is where the blood flow to the heart is restricted, leading to damage of the heart muscle. Coronary artery disease is usually due to atherosclerosis – the thickening of blood vessel walls resulting from fatty deposits. The risk of this is much higher if you eat a high-fat diet, have high cholesterol or are obese.

Happily, the death rate from this disease has fallen dramatically in recent years with better education about not smoking, eating healthily and exercising regularly.

Cancer

Cancer is a disease that makes cells overmultiply and cause damage in the body. Since there are so many different cancers, at the moment there is no single cause that has been established. However, the World Cancer Research Fund is now recommending – as part of its cancer prevention action plan – that participants perform up to one hour's exercise every day.

Are you really fat?

Having talked about what and where fat is, the next question to consider is whether you *really* are fat. The trouble with people who become obsessed with what they eat every day and how much they should be exercising every hour is that they can often have a distorted view of how fat they really are. This kind of thinking in its severest form can lead to compulsive eating disorders. At the other end of the scale, people who are over-fat can often be very resistant to admitting that they eat too much. Food is a great comforter and overeating is habit forming. Therefore, when undertaking a programme of change, it is important to be realistic. As with many things in life, the middle way is often better than the extremes.

Take a realistic look at your body and start to think about how you can do the best for it. Consider how your body would look if it carried less fat and if it was toned with the muscles showing through, instead of wishing your legs were longer, which you can't change, or just that you weighed less, which is misleading.

'Fat' versus 'weight'
The amount of body fat you carry is much more important than your weight according to scales. The body mass index (BMI) is one commonly used way of assessing whether a person holds too much body fat in relation to their height and shape. The waist-to-hips ratio rating (see box, right) is another.

Many men tend to accumulate excess body fat around their middles, while women have a tendency to accumulate fat around the thighs and hips. The waist-to-hips ratio rating focuses on the fat in this area of the body only, independent of total body fat. The lower the waist-to-hip ratio rating, the healthier you are. A high score can be associated with heart disease and other obesity-linked conditions (see 'Fat storage', page 13). In men, the score should be 0.95 or less, in women an acceptable score is 0.85 or less.

If your score is above these levels, don't panic, but instead use it as an impetus to start your fat-burning regime. Being too fat does carry risks and it is worth being aware of them and making the changes so that you can reduce any danger to your long-term health.

Focusing on fat
Fat is not only a visual thing. You know yourself, from the feel of your body in your clothes, whether you are carrying too much fat.

Don't confuse the 'fat feeling'

We all have times when we *feel* fat. This can often cause us to feel depressed. Be aware, however, that it is easy to focus on how being 'fat' makes us unhappy because it is so visual. It may in fact be that the way you look is not the real issue. If this feeling occurs too regularly, try to look beyond the obvious and see if anything else is troubling you. If other areas of your life need attention, focus on these for a while and leave the body issue aside. When you go back to it you may see yourself differently.

We all have areas where we tend to accumulate fat. Women often mention the back of the arms, as a place that carries fat and men notice the fat that sits on the side of the hips – commonly called 'love handles'.

The fat-burner workout programme in Chapter 4 will certainly provide opportunities to tone specific areas (see also pages 112–113). However, just as you cannot dictate where fat accumulates first, you cannot dictate where it will come off. Fat is stored all over the body and it reduces in the body in a similar pattern. So, the fat that went on last will most probably come off first – and you may not even be aware of where that was.

Calculate your waist-to-hips ratio rating

1 Take a tape measure and measure your waist. Your waistline runs approximately around where your navel is. Pull the tape so that it fits snugly around your bare skin, but don't distort the skin by pulling too tight! Note the reading.

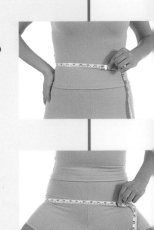

2 To measure your hips, bend your knees slightly. Now wrap the tape measure just around where the tops of the thighs meet the hips, i.e. where you bend naturally. Pull the tape so that it sits snugly and note the measurement.

3 To calculate the rating, divide your waist measurement by your hip measurement. For example, if your waist measures 69cm (27in) and your hips 91cm (36in), then 69 ÷ 91 (27 ÷ 36) = 0.75.

In **men**, the score should be **0.95 or less**.
In **women** an acceptable score is **0.85 or less**.

How do you lose body fat?

Earlier sections in this chapter have now established that it is a good idea not to be fat, and have encouraged you to consider how fat you personally are. So, assuming that you have fat to lose – how do you go about it?

Despite all kinds of diets, equipment, potions, pills and creams, there are really only three ways to change your body shape:
▶ Eat less
▶ Exercise more
▶ Undergo surgery!

Eat less

Eating less does not have to mean starving yourself. It really means eating regular meals – as many as three to six per day – combined with making sensible food choices (see page 36).

Choosing healthier foods really means opting for foods that provide a good source of nutrients and roughage. Plentiful vitamins and minerals keep your system in good condition, while fibre-rich foods aid the digestion. The problem with much of today's shop-bought processed food, and with the food offered in many cafés and fast-food outlets, is that it is often very low in nutritional content. Such foods tend to have a high content of fat, sugar and salt. This makes them tasty and moreish but of little nutritional value to the body. If you consume large quantities of this type of food, not only do you deplete your body's nutritional supplies but you will also gain weight.

In contrast, eating lots more natural foods – fresh fruit, vegetables and whole grains – provides the vitamins and minerals the body needs. These foods are filling so you can eat well and feel full without piling on excessive calories. They are also low in fat and salt, and you can use them to create endless tasty, appetizing recipes.

As you make better food choices you will find your body storing less fat and your slimmer self beginning to emerge.

Exercise more

When you exercise your body uses up calories to provide energy. The more energy you use up, the fewer calories are left to be stored in the body (see page 24). If you regularly use up lots of calories through exercise, you will find your body becomes leaner, with fewer calories being stored as body fat.

There is also an additional benefit to exercise. With regular exercise your body will build up muscle. Muscle needs calories for its upkeep and therefore even fewer calories are stored. Thus, both exercise and the build-up of muscle boost your metabolism by increasing the rate at which calories are burned. The result is that not only do you look leaner but you also begin to appear stronger, shapelier and fitter looking.

Undergo surgery!

Some people consider this option as a way of changing their shape. While it may work for women who want to enlarge their breasts or for men who want to change the shape of their nose, sadly surgery is not an effective way to lose body fat in the long term.

When you undergo liposuction the fat cells are vacuumed out from beneath the skin to leave you with less fat and looking slimmer. But ask yourself this question: how long can it possibly last?

If the reason you had excess fat in the first place was from overeating and underexercising, then your body's process of laying

down fat is not going to stop just because you have got rid of a few fat cells. If you continue to take in more calories than your body uses, your body will simply create new fat cells to store the excess. These fat cells will then get created elsewhere in the body and you may end up with unslightly lumps somewhere else! Unless you change your eating and exercising habits, the potential for laying down more fat remains. It would be far better to try to think of this programme as a kick start to a long-term health plan that will keep on working for longer than the results of the surgery option.

If you do not change your habits you will have spent lots of money and undergone lots of discomfort to gain a figure that will not last! Spend a few months getting your activity and eating plan into action and it can be something that can stay with you for life.

Comparison of weight loss methods

✗ Unnatural intervention	versus	✔ Healthy eating regime and fitness programme
✗ Expensive and short-lived	versus	✔ Cheap and lasting
✗ Surgery	versus	✔ Regular exercise
✗ Fad diets	versus	✔ Sensible eating
✗ Fat-busting pills, potions and creams	versus	✔ Healthy, natural choices

2 Working out

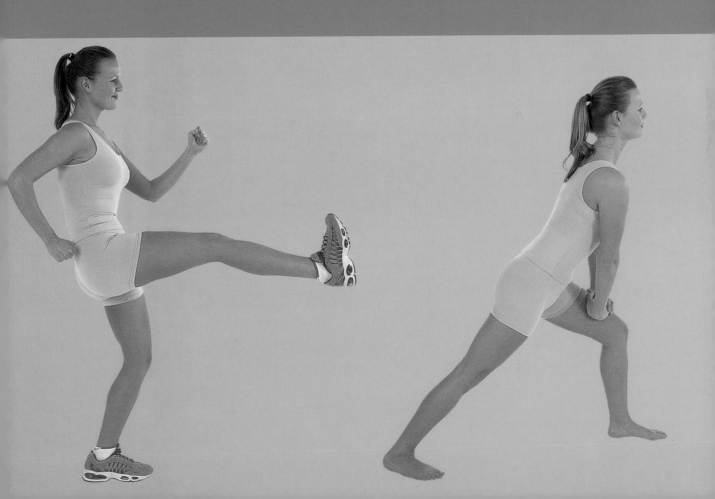

Losing body fat through exercise

You now know that exercise is a great idea for many reasons; you also know that exercise is one of the keys to reducing your body fat. But how exactly do you do it?

When it comes to fat loss there is one very simple equation that is all you need to remember:

▶ If you eat *more* energy (i.e. calories) than you need and don't use it up through exercise, you will store the excess as body fat, i.e. you become fatter.

▶ If you eat *less* energy than you need and exercise more, your body will use up stored fat to provide the necessary energy, i.e. you become slimmer.

So, the only solution is to eat less and exercise more (see box, top right).

Now that you can see how simple the process is, exactly what should you be doing in order to burn fat? The issues involved are the type of exercise (see page 26), the intensity of the workout (see page 28) and the role of the metabolism (see page 30).

The benefits of exercise

Exercising regularly will not only burn fat but also improve other areas of your health. When you exercise regularly, you will notice that you will:

▶ Increase the strength of your heart, lungs and muscles – keeping them healthy.

▶ Gain energy.

▶ Build muscles, which require more calories to maintain and so increase the metabolism.

▶ Improve your posture with toned muscles.

▶ Gain a good-looking body and confidence.

▶ Develop better drinking and eating habits. When you exercise, you become more aware of your body and start to look after it better. Your body also starts to crave the 'right' kinds of food.

▶ Sweat as you exercise – this encourages thirst and replacement of lost fluids, and allows the body to cleanse itself by eliminating unwanted products. Drinking water regularly helps the body systems and keeps the bladder healthy.

▶ Boost your mood and feelings of wellbeing and ward off depression.

As you work out and clear your head you will feel refreshed, de-stressed and more able to face life's challenges.

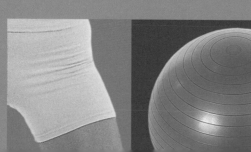
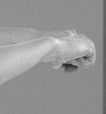
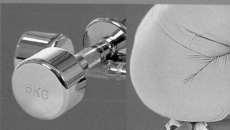

The full figures for fat loss

Consider the following facts and apply them to your own fat-burning workout programme:
▶ To lose weight (body fat) you need to burn calories

500g (1lb) of fat = 3500 calories

▶ If a 63.5kg (140lb) runner, for example, burns 100 calories per mile then she needs to run 35 miles to burn off 500g (1lb).

▶ If you run 3 miles four times per week you will have burned 1200 calories that week. So in just under three weeks you will have lost 500g (1lb) of body fat!

Change your eating habits:
▶ If you do without your 250-calorie chocolate bar and run 2½ miles you will create a calorie deficit of 500 calories. Do this every day and you will have a deficit of 3500 calories in one week!

Muscle-strengthening also helps:
▶ As you exercise, you build muscle. For every 500g (1lb) of muscle gained you will use an extra 50 calories! You will increase your metabolism, burning more calories even when resting. It is not just how many calories you burn while exercising that counts.

Visible results of fat loss

As your body fat stores are reduced you will notice a:
▶ Smoothing of your skin – cells beneath are less bobbly.

▶ Change in body shape – fewer stored fat pockets mean a smoothing out of your shape.

▶ Feeling of being less heavy – you are carrying less fat around.

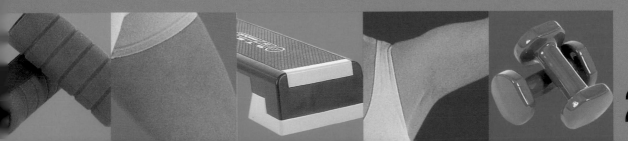

Types of fat-burning exercise

Most exercise is either aerobic or anaerobic. The terms refer to the energy system the body uses when doing different types of exercise. The two types of exercise make different demands on the body.

Aerobic exercise

Aerobic exercise essentially means 'with air', which means that the body uses oxygen to metabolise stored fat into energy. Aerobic exercise is characterized by the fact that you would be using large muscle groups rhythmically for a period of 20 minutes or longer. At this point the body needs to metabolize its stored energy into the bloodstream in order to keep the activity going.

As you continue to work through and beyond the 20-minute period you have the satisfaction of knowing your body will then be delving into your fat stores to keep your body moving. So you are literally using up stored fat!

Bear in mind also, that as your body gets used to exercising regularly in this mode it switches into this mode sooner, so that you may well be metabolising fat after 15 rather than 20 minutes.

What aerobic exercise involves

▶ Different types of rhythmic exercise using large muscle groups, for example running, cycling, swimming, rowing, cross-country skiing.

▶ Relatively medium exertion intensity – if you are working too hard you won't be able to keep going for 20 minutes.

▶ Rhythmic work into which the body can relax and where the muscles or limbs aren't overstressed.

▶ Variety of movement (or if that isn't possible, for example when running, then at least a variety of view), so that you're not too bored to keep going for at least 20 minutes.

▶ Your breathing should be regular and not gasping but the heart will be pumping relatively hard. You should be able to maintain some form of conversation, while exercising aerobically. If you can't, then the activity becomes anaerobic.

Anaerobic exercise

Exercise that is not aerobic, such as muscle-strengthening, is often classed as anaerobic. This means that as you lift weights or perform stomach curl-ups, for example, you are using glycogen, rather than fat, as the primary fuel for energy. Instead of eating into your fat stores, you are using the fuel already available in your muscles. When you run out of this fuel your muscles will ache and you will need to stop. This type of exercise still has an important place in your fat-burning routine however.

Remember that:
▶ If you are trying to lose body fat, then muscle-strengthening is important because the more muscle your body has, the more calories will be needed to maintain it. Therefore instead of your body storing excess calories as fat, it will utilize those calories to maintain your muscle mass.

▶ Extra muscle will mean your posture is improved, you will move with more energy and you have a more defined shape.

After 20 minutes of any aerobic exercise (see box below) you are using your fat supplies for exercising. However, since your ultimate goal is body fat loss, and therefore to burn calories (to get your deficit of 3500 calories per week, for example), add in some higher intensity work such as muscle-strengthening when you exercise. The harder you work, the more calories are needed; even if some of those calories comes from stored carbohydrates it is still going towards your total deficit.

In the 30-day fat-burning workout programme in Chapter 4 you will find some great ways to increase and vary the intensity of your exercise. Not only will this diversify your workouts but it will also burn even more calories.

Aerobic activities and their energy (calorie) use per hour

▶ Aerobic classes 350 kcals

▶ Cross-country skiing 500 kcals

▶ Cycling 400 kcals

▶ Dancing 300 kcals

▶ Fast swimming 500 kcals

▶ Fast walking 250 kcals

▶ Football 450 kcals

▶ Jogging 500 kcals

▶ Rope skipping 450 kcals

▶ Cleaning windows 350 kcals

How hard should you work out?

To burn the optimum amount of body fat, you should be doing a low- to medium-intensity exercise for at least 20 minutes. When you exercise aerobically in this way, fat is used as the primary fuel. The chart below explains the stages of fuel consumption that your body goes through when you exercise.

Start the exercise clock

0–10 minutes
Carbohydrates (sugars) already stored in the muscle are used as your body begins to move. These come from the food and drink you have consumed today and are adequate for the initial energy demand at this stage.

10–20 minutes
Carbohydrates in the working muscles are now running low. Fat and carbohydrates from stored supplies are broken down and begin to be released into the bloodstream, ready to be picked up and used by the muscles. Breathing and heart rate will both have increased so as to supply more oxygen to the working body.

At 20 minutes
Fat is increasingly metabolized from storage for energy. Carbohydrates from the liver are utilized and the blood now has plenty of circulating fat, sugar and oxygen to feed the muscles and help release more energy from storage.

20–60 minutes – maximum fat-burning time
Your body is now using the aerobic system to supply fuel, breaking down fats and transforming them into energy to keep the muscles working. As long as there is enough oxygen coming in – via regular breathing – then fat is the primary fuel keeping the body going. It is during this period that fat-burning is maximized.

Over one hour
If the intensity of the exercise increases, carbohydrates stored as body fat will be the preferred fuel. If the exercise goes on beyond two hours, protein may well be used to supply the energy required.

Determining the intensity level of your workout

You can use different levels of intensity to challenge your body, but how do you know when you are exercising at which level? How do you know if you are even in your aerobic zone?

The target heart rate (THR) can help you determine how hard you are working. This method is used to estimate the intensity level someone is working at. It uses the heart rate and percentages of it to calculate two figures, which give the parameters for hard work and lower-level work (see box below).

If your heart rate does not reach the lower parameter you are not working hard enough for the exercise to be aerobic, i.e. fat-burning and you will not be losing fat. If you stray too far out of the THR zone you may find that the exercise becomes anaerobic.

Another simpler way to tell whether you are exercising aerobically or anaerobically is simply to check whether you can carry on a conversation as you exercise. (If you are cycling alone try singing to yourself.)

Calculating your target heart rate (THR)

1. Calculate your *maximum* heart rate by subtracting your age from 220.

2. Calculate 55 and 85 per cent of this figure to give you two parameters between which your heart rate should operate in order to be fairly sure you are exercising aerobically:
55 per cent would be a low-intensity workout
85 per cent would be a high-intensity workout

If you are working below 55 per cent, you are not working hard enough for the exercise to be aerobic i.e. fat-burning. If you work above or around 85 per cent, it will be anaerobic and unsustainable for any length of time.

For example the approximate maximum heart rate of a 40-year-old beginner exerciser would be 220–40 = 180 beats per minute (bpm). The parameters for his heart rate are:
55% x 180 = 99
85% x 180 = 153
i.e. THR = 99–153bpm

This beginner's heart rate should be between 99 and 153bpm when he checks his pulse (see box below). As he is a beginner he should initially aim to reach the lower figure, and build up to the 20 minutes. As his experience and strength increases he might well start to train at the higher end of this spectrum.

Checking your pulse

1. To discover your resting pulse check your heart rate in the morning before getting up. Using two fingers together, press down lightly on the thumb side of the upturned wrist of the other hand to feel your pulse. Start the timer and count the number of beats felt by your fingers for 60 seconds.

2. To determine your heart rate while working out, stop momentarily mid-session and take your pulse in the same way for just six seconds, again counting the first beat as zero. Multiply this figure by ten to calculate the number of beats per minute.

The role of the metabolism in burning fat

As we have seen, exercise is responsible for burning calories but the metabolism also has a part to play in fat-burning.

Regular exercise achieves several things:
▶ You build muscle tissue, which requires energy for its upkeep.
▶ You eat regularly because you are hungry.
▶ Your body becomes used to a regular cycle: a regular input of food, which regularly gets converted to energy, which is used up in activity.
▶ On completion of an exercise session, your body burns calories at an elevated rate for several hours afterwards.
▶ With more muscles and more energy your desire to be active increases.

All these factors mean that your body uses up energy at a higher rate than the body of someone who does not exercise or eat regularly. This plays a key role in keeping body fat at a good level.

Metabolic myths

Many myths surround the concept of the metabolism. For example it is often assumed that overweight people have a slow metabolism. This just isn't true. It is people who severely restrict their food intake who end up slowing down their metabolism (see page 36). People who overeat actually have a faster metabolism.

Thanks to studies from both sides of the Atlantic, it has now been scientifically proven that fat people have a faster metabolism. Eating large amounts of food regularly means the body has to work hard to digest the food and keeps the metabolism raised. Even at rest, the fat person expends more energy than the thin person does. Not only this, but fat people can also have very strong muscles, for example they need very strong leg muscles to carry all that weight around. The problem faced by the fat person is not their metabolism, but the fact that all those consumed calories don't get used up and therefore get stored as increasing amounts of body fat.

Raising your metabolism

You can increase your metabolism yourself, and this should in fact be your aim to aid fat-burning.

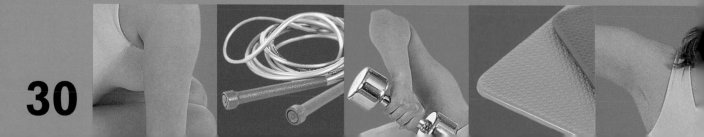

How to build muscle

In order to build muscle you have to work the muscle. When you are doing an aerobic workout the work must be prolonged enough so that the heart is really having to work to pump the blood around the body. You should notice two things:

▶ you will feel your heart pumping

▶ you will be breathing hard, but you should still be able to carry on a conversation

It is this kind of work though, that will challenge the heart and get it to become stronger and more efficient.

When you do weighted workouts, make sure the weights are heavy enough. Start gradually so that you don't injure yourself, but as you feel yourself getting stronger, then increase the weight so that you feel challenged after eight to ten repetitions of the exercise.

However, it needs strenuous exercise on a regular basis – that is, three to four times per week.

Studies show that people who perform this level of exercise have an increased metabolism, even when they sleep. The exercise does need to be vigorous and prolonged (for at least 45 minutes), however, and it is suggested that the exercise needs to be done at least every other day to keep the metabolism raised. One of the key ways to increase the metabolism is to increase your muscle mass. It is often assumed that as we get older our metabolism slows down and this is why we naturally gain weight as we age. This is not strictly true. What does happen is that we tend to lose muscle mass as we get older, which slows the rate down. The average adult loses 2.75kg (6lb) of muscle every ten years, through reduced activity and fewer demands on the body. Every time we lose muscle we decrease our resting metabolic rate and decrease our need for calories. So the opposite applies – build muscle to increase your metabolism.

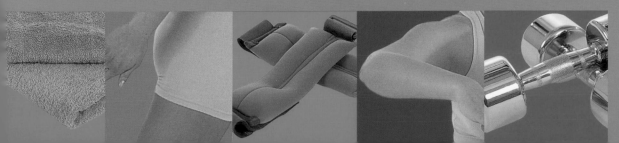

Developing a fat-burning programme

You will, by now, be starting to understand a little of what needs to go into a true fat-burning workout. A foolproof plan needs several elements to cover all the aspects of keeping the body healthy and hungry and burning those calories.

In Chapter 4 you will find a full 30-day programme that will guide you through a month of solid fat-burning training. However, with the information in all the other chapters you should be able to vary this routine and put together your own kind of fitness programme, for future use.

Starting out

As you start to build your programme bear in mind the basic principles. It should include the following components.

Cardiovascular exercise

Progressive and varied sessions of cardiovascular exercise (CV), building in length to at least 20 minutes, are required. This type of workout will directly burn body fat and significant amounts of calories. It will also have the added benefit of strengthening your heart and lungs, making you more energetic.

Proper warming-up and cooling-down

The warm-up will prepare your body and mind for its activity, while the cooling-down stretches at the end of your workout will return your muscles to their pre-exercise state and prevent injury (see pages 48–51).

Muscle-strengthening work

Exercises specifically designed to help strengthen muscles will use up calories, while the toned muscles will provide a strong firm frame that moves with ease and confidence and supports the spine with strong abdominals.

Regular exercise

No exercise programme will work unless you do it regularly. The recommendation for fat-burning is to exercise every day, hence the programme in Chapter 4 is ideally to be followed over 30 consecutive days. Exercising every day in this way allows the body a 24-hour recovery period between fitness sessions, which is enough time to rest your muscles. If you cannot exercise every day, exercising every other day is the next best option.

Be prepared

Now that you are committed to starting training, ensure that nothing is going to hold you back. A fat-burning programme will not work unless it is done regularly – at least three times per week and preferably every day to be the most effective. Most of the workouts in the 30-day programme that starts on page 52 should take you between 35 and 45 minutes, which includes a good 20–30 minutes of CV exercise for maximum fat-burning. So before you start do a quick check:

Have you got the right shoes?
Check that you have cross-training or running shoes for your CV work. Shoes should not have had more than 16 weeks of wear and should be in good, bouncy condition. If they are not in good nick – buy new ones. After all you don't want your fab fat-burning routine to be held back, just as you are getting into the swing of it, by shin splints or blisters.

Have you got the right gear?
You are going to be breaking sweat with this programme and you may well be out in all weathers, so get the gear: rainproofs, gloves, changes of T-shirts and kagoule. Women need good sports bras and underwear.

Have you checked with your doctor?
It is always wise to double check with a doctor who knows you well, before you embark on any home fitness programme. Tell them what you intend so that if they have any concerns about your blood pressure or your ability to complete such a programme, they can advise you accordingly.

Exercise time is time for *you*

▶ Don't miss a session because you think you haven't got time.

▶ For every hour you spend exercising, you will get back double in terms of the energy levels you will have for the rest of the day.

▶ Remember that time spent exercising will take you away from the stresses and excitements of your day and allow you time to think, relax, focus or be creative.

Have you told friends and family?
A fat-burning programme takes dedication so start to warn those closest to you that you may be unavailable from time to time – or maybe just a little later to arrive – in order to fit in your exercise sessions.

Have you told your diary?
There is no single correct time to exercise – it really comes down to when you think you can best fit a session in. Most people who exercise regularly tend to do their routine in the morning so that it gets done and is out of the way, but the time of day at which you exercise really makes no difference to the body. Pick a time that suits you and you are able to stick to. Put it in your diary as an appointment and cancel it only in dire circumstances!

33

34

3 Nutrition and diet

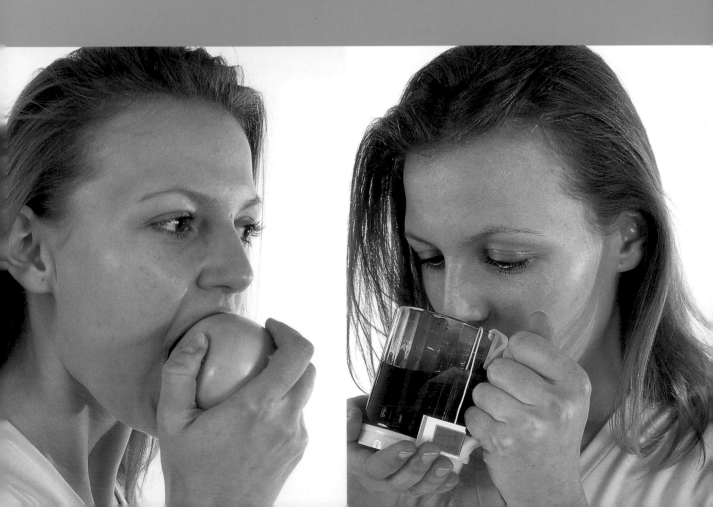

How to eat sensibly

As with many aspects of health nowadays, there is much conflicting advice around on what to eat and how to eat it. These and the following pages set out the latest advice on eating that is available.

Eat little and often

It is important when you are trying to burn body fat – and lead a healthy existence – that you drink plenty of water (see box, page 36) and eat regularly. If you go for long periods without eating you will not have the energy you need to conduct your daily business easily. Regular eating will keep your blood sugar levels steady and your mood elevated.

People who restrict their food intake too much are frustrating themselves on two accounts:
▶ When exercising you want to burn body fat with cardiovascular (CV) exercise. As you continue to exercise with oxygen present (aerobic exercise) you utilize your fat stores to provide energy. But don't forget that when you exercise aerobically you use a combination of glycogen (muscle fuel from carbohydrates) and fat. Without carbohydrates to get the process going you won't burn fat.
▶ If you restrict your food intake too acutely, the body acts as though there may be starvation on the horizon and starts to conserve body fat. It also starts to conserve energy and slow down the metabolism. So you will find it increasingly hard to lose weight. Thus, if you try to lose weight simply by restricting calorie intake alone (i.e. rigid dieting)

you will move less because you have less energy and your body composition will start to change. With less muscle and more body fat it will become increasingly difficult to lose weight and life will become distinctly dreary.

Eat low in fat

When you overeat, it doesn't matter whether you have eaten fat, carbohydrate or protein – the excess will still be stored under the skin as fat. While some fat in the diet is beneficial, there are two very good reasons to eat a diet that is relatively low in fat.

Firstly, the fat that we eat has far more calories (the term used to describe the amount of heat generated by the body from food) per gram than protein or carbohydrates:
▶ Carbohydrate:
4 calories per gram
▶ Protein:
4 calories per gram
▶ Fat:
9 calories per gram

So, if you are trying to restrict your calories, remember you can eat more carbohydrates and protein for less calories than fats. In other words, you can eat more plates of vegetables before clocking up 300 calories than packets of crisps, which are high in fat.

Types of fat in the diet

A certain amount of fat is essential in our diets to keep us healthy and provide as with some important vitamins. In particular we need small amounts of the essential fatty acids (EFAs), which the body cannot manufacture itself and which are vital for a healthy heart, blood and brain.

▶ **Saturated fats:** These are usually solid at room temperature and tend to come from animal sources – the fat on meat, butter, lard and cheese. Vegetable sources of saturated fat are coconut butter and palm oil. High quantities of saturated fats are 'hidden' in many fast and processed foods, e.g. in biscuits, pastries, pies and ice cream. A diet high in this type of fat increases the most harmful form of cholesterol, the low-density lipoprotein (LDL), in the blood, which increases the risk of heart disease.

▶ **Polyunsaturated fats:** These contain the EFAs we require. Good sources are fresh nuts and seeds and their oils (such as corn, safflower, sunflower, walnut and soya bean oils and spreads), green leafy vegetables, and oily fish (such as kippers, herring, sardines, tuna, salmon, mackerel) and fish supplements. These fats lower the body's total cholesterol, so are better for you than saturated fats. However, the 'good' cholesterol, high-density lipoprotein (HDL) needs to be kept high, so you still don't want too many of these fats.

▶ **Monounsaturated fats:** Olive oil is our main source of monounsaturated fat; others are rapeseed oil, peanuts and avocados. These fats lower the LDL in the blood and should not decrease the HDL too much – so these are the preferable fats to take. Try and replace some of the saturated fat in your diet with monounsaturated fat.

Secondly, a diet too high in fat, particularly saturated fat, is known to contribute to coating the arteries and veins and thus restricting their width, which can then lead to heart problems.

Eat lots of vegetables and fruit

The best rule to abide by is: every time you have a plate of food try to make sure there is some fruit or vegetables on it. Vegetables and fruit contain important vitamins, minerals and other nutrients, so they should be the first priority. Try to ensure these make up the majority of your diet by making them the largest portion on your plate. A diet rich in fruit and vegetables is thought to help guard against carcinogens (substances that cause cancer), arthritis and many other illnesses including heart disease.

Drink plenty of water

▶ Try to drink at least eight to ten glasses of water per day. Dehydration can occur without you becoming aware of it. In fact, if you are thirsty, you are already dehydrated.

▶ Dehydration can effect your posture (by plumping up the discs between the vertabrae), your energy levels and your hunger levels. Dehydration also lowers the metabolism by two to three per cent.

▶ Try different types of water and add a little fresh fruit juice for a quick refresher after a workout.

▶ If you keep a bottle of water handy throughout your day and sip rather than glug back a whole pint or half-litre at once – you won't be rushing to the toilet every five minutes!

Fruit and vegetables are also great foods when it comes to fat loss. They supply excellent energy in the form of complex carbohydrates and are low in both calories and fat. This means you can eat more of them than of other foods and so feel comfortably full and satisfied without consuming excess calories.

In addition to this, most fruit is easy to carry with you as a handy snack for any time of day. Bananas in particular are a really fast energy source, so keep one handy when you exercise. Don't forget canned and frozen fruits and vegetables are equally good and convenient for providing nutrients and carbohydrates.

Eat whole grains
Whole wheat and rice products provide the complex carbohydrates the body needs to keep the blood sugar levels balanced. Too many refined grains can cause a surge in blood sugar levels followed by a feeling of low energy when the effects wear off. So try to include whole grain breads, pasta or rice on your plate once a day.

Avoid too much sugar
Not only does sugar provide 'empty' calories (calories with no nutrients), an excess of which may be stored as body fat, it also upsets your body's blood sugar levels. Rapid rises in blood sugar cause the body to produce higher levels of insulin, the hormone that helps regulate blood sugar levels. Long-term overconsumption of sugar results in a permanently raised level of insulin in the blood, which in turns leads to health problems such as diabetes. Therefore it is best to try to keep your intake of sugar to a minimum.

Handy snacks for exercising

▶ Dried fruit such as apricots, apple slices, raisins, banana chips, prunes

▶ High fruit-content bars

▶ Low-fat fruity cereal bars

▶ Bananas

▶ Kiwi fruit – with the top sliced off and eaten like a boiled egg

Watch your salt intake

A high salt intake has been linked with stomach cancer and is thought to raise blood pressure so keep its use to a minimum. Add small amounts to cooking (only half the amount stated by recipes) and do not add salt directly to food after it has been prepared.

Limit your consumption of alcohol

While some studies suggest a glass of red wine may be beneficial to blood pressure, there is not much good in alcohol – particularly for the fat-burner. We all know it is a great relaxant and socializer and it is impractical to suggest you should never touch another drop – but remember the maxim: as little as possible!

Alcohol, of any description, does three devastating things for the fat-burner:
▶ It turns off your appetite switch. When you drink you cease to notice what you are putting in your body. As you become influenced by the alcohol it can turn off your natural 'I have had enough' switch so that you don't notice you are full and you keep eating. This leaves you feeling ill and stuffed, and significantly overloads your calories.
▶ It turns on your fat storing cells. Unlike fat, carbohydrates or proteins, alcohol is not used by the body for any healthy processes. It is regarded as a toxin by the body, which tries to expel it. The sugar that comes from alcohol, however, is stored as fat if not used up immediately. In addition, it primes your cells to store more fat!
▶ It turns off your will power. If you have spent days working on your fat-burning programme don't blow your progress with one evening of overindulgence. After a few glasses of alcohol you might start to think you don't care if you don't stick to your eating /exercising programme any more. The next morning you *will* care and you'll wish you hadn't done it!

Keep a food diary

Many people are fairly unaware of what they put into their bodies on a day-to-day basis. Busy lives carry on regardless and often it is hard to remember whether you had three biscuits with your coffee or an extra sandwich at the end of that meeting! Scientific research has found that many overweight people simply underestimate what they eat, or forget to take account of the calories in drink or snacks.

The point at which you start the fat-burner workout programme is a good time to take a look at your eating patterns. Following the example set out below, record what, when and how much you eat for between five and seven days, making sure you include a weekend. Then use the guidelines and analysis to assess your eating habits and identify any possible downfalls that may be lurking.

Guidelines

Record *all* food and drink that you consume over the five- to seven-day period.

▶ Try to be as specific as you can, giving amounts such as cups, grams, ounces, litres, tablespoonfuls, pints, etc.

▶ List whether the meal was homemade or bought ready-made.

▶ List the way that food was cooked, for example boiled, fried, grilled.

▶ Record the time that food was eaten – this may give you some pointers for future fat-burning.

▶ List whether you ate in a restaurant or at home.

▶ Remember to include the type and quantity of milk and sugar used in drinks and butter or margarine used on your bread.

Saturday 29 June

Breakfast 07:30: *At home*
1 piece of wholemeal bread, toasted, scraping of low-fat spread and 1 teaspoon of honey.
1 glass of apple juice
Cup of tea made with skimmed milk.

Lunch 13:00: *Bought from bagel shop*
1 plain bagel filled with 2 teaspoons full-fat cream cheese, ham, tomatoes, cucumber and lettuce.
celery and carrot sticks *brought from home*.

Dinner 20:00: *At home*
1 grilled chicken breast, 4 steamed new potatoes, selection of steamed vegetables.
1 low-fat fruit yogurt
1 glass of white wine (125ml glass)

Snacks:
2 digestive biscuits
1 apple
1 packet of plain crisps
¼ pint of skimmed milk for cups of tea

Analysis of your food diary

Look back over the last five to seven days and ask yourself the following questions, to which the answers should be 'yes'!

1 Have I eaten regularly? (Ideally every four hours)

2 Have I chosen my snacks well (e.g. fruits, vegetables, nuts, hummus and pitta bread, as opposed to processed sugary snacks such as chocolate bars, biscuits and crisps)?

3 Have I often eaten starchy food (e.g. bread, pasta, breakfast cereals, rice, potatoes)?

4 Have I often eaten protein foods (e.g. fish, meat, chicken, dairy products, vegetarian products)?

5 Have I drunk water regularly throughout each day?

6 Have I eaten more reduced-fat than full-fat dairy products (e.g. skimmed milk and low-fat yogurt)?

7 Have I eaten fried food less often?

8 Have I managed to eat five portions of fruit and vegetables daily? (One serving equates to 40g/1½oz of a vegetable or one piece of fruit or a small glass of fresh juice.)

9 Have I eaten out less than twice per week (including café visits)?

10 When I have eaten out, have I resisted the temptation to overindulge?

11 Have I consumed less than seven units per alcohol per week? (one unit equates to 125ml/4 fl oz glass of wine, 300ml/½ pint of beer or one measure of spirits)

12 Have I eaten enough so that I have not felt hungry or cold?

13 Have I eaten carefully enough that I have not felt bloated?

If the answer to all of the above questions is **'yes' – you are doing pretty well! If** some of the answers are **'no'** then **try to work on these aspects** of your dietary behaviour. Start on the fitness programme in the following chapter and try to change your **'no'** eating habits around. Take this quiz again and aim, by the end of this book to make all the answers **'yes'**!

Eating and exercising

Eating and exercising are your partners in success when it comes to fat burning and shape changing. Dieting alone can cause a loss of muscle tone which not only reduces your shape, but your ability to use up calories too. When you exercise you need to eat well to support the body as it rises to the physical challenge. As you exercise and eat well you will feel full of energy and full of resolve to keep up your regime.

Dieting

You can use this book with your own diet if you want to. Many different diets have been put forward as the key to weight loss, but some people have more success with one type rather than another. As yet, there have been no conclusive studies that prove one diet to be unfailingly more successful than any another. Often, all we have to go on is media hype and myth-like stories of celebrity weight loss. There are many types of diet that can be followed – from no-combination diets to protein-only or carbohydrate-loading – and it really comes down to which suits you personally.

Remember that the diet you choose needs to be practical. You stand a better chance of sticking to it if it fits into your normal life. How practical – and how healthy, for example, is a diet that involves living on only grapefruit for 20 days? Is the diet complicated? If it involves lots of soaking of pulses the night before, or buying obscure products from healthfood stores, will it take up too much time or money to be practical? Make sure the diet uses a good range of normal foods.

Eating and working out

Stick to the following golden rules for eating and working out and you will be able to combine healthy eating with fat-burning exercise to achieve the look and shape you want.

Eat before and after working out

Eat at least 90 minutes before exercising to give your body enough fuel and to avoid indigestion. Eat afterwards to replace used energy.

Have breakfast

Your body needs a kick start in the morning to restart the metabolism so don't slow it down by denying it. If you don't believe the benefits try this: on Tuesday and Thursday treat yourself to a healthy start of porridge and fruit juice. See if you don't feel better than on Monday and Wednesday when you have nothing.

Keep nutritious snacks handy

If you run out of fruit, vegetable sticks, nuts, dried fruit and rice cakes and you are left with only chocolate biscuits you'll be forced to eat them! So try and always provide yourself with a healthy alternative to the wrong kind of snack foods.

Stop to think differently about food

When you are working out regularly – try to think of food as a source of energy rather than as the enemy. Ask yourself whether the food you are about to eat is nutritional and energy giving, or is it just 'empty' calories? It may sound obvious but if you keep asking yourself these questions you will start to make better food choices, more often.

Eat little and often

Not eating for lengthy periods slows down the metabolism. It is recommended that you eat four to six small meals (which means about every four hours) per day. This helps to keep your energy and mood levels high.

Being 'naughty'

If you really must indulge by having that chocolate bar, then make sure you eat it after your workout. Your metabolism will be at its highest after exercising so that is the best time to eat unhealthy snacks

Power snack

Before a long meeting, a physical pursuit or a stressful situation you know is coming up, 'power snack' on rice cakes, oats, rusks, wholemeal toast, fruit, yogurt and honey, nuts, sunflower bars (available from healthfood stores) and even certain baby foods! If you know you'll have a really early start in the morning then eat some pasta, rice or popcorn the night before to help set you up.

The right diet for you

Choose a diet that:
▶ Uses foods you like.

▶ Uses varied foods and doesn't focus on just one food.

▶ Allows you to eat carbohydrates, proteins and some fats. Despite all the hype, the body has evolved utilizing all these elements, so the chances are that in the right amounts, they are not going to do you any harm.

▶ Gives you three to four meals per day. As we have already seen (page 36), radical cutting back will not give you enough energy to do the workout side of this programme and too little food will slow you down and reduce your ability to build muscle.

Stay hydrated

Drink eight to ten glasses of water per day – ideally 1 litre (1¾ pints) of bottled water – and sip regularly during and after exercise. You need 'sports drinks' only if your exercise session has exceeded 90 minutes, but try 50/50 fruit juice and water for a great pick-me-up.

Avoid alcohol

Alcohol dehydrates the body and provides 'empty' calories that you will have to use up. It can also leave you with a nasty hangover, one of the biggest de-motivators when it comes to exercising. If you have overdone it drink lots of water for the next 48 hours.

▶ **Get set to go**

▶ **The daily programme**

▶ **Maintaining your new figure**

4 The 30-day fat-burning programme

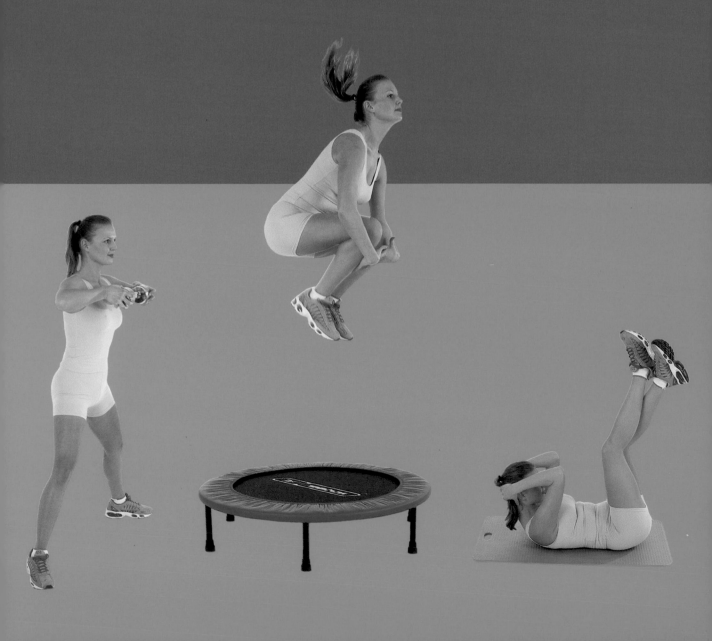

Get set to go

The previous chapters have established some very sound principles about what it takes to burn fat with exercise and eating. Basically, the more intense the activity, the more fat you burn (even though the percentage of fat burned continues to drop), the harder your muscles have to work, the more calories you burn – remember weight loss is calories in versus calories out – so get using up calories! Work faster and harder – that way you'll get through more miles, more mountains and more calories in the 1 hour or whatever time you have available.

How to use this programme

▶ In general, the programme comprises a progressively challenging set of exercises for each of the 30 days. Most days include some cardiovascular exercise for direct body-fat burning or some anaerobic exercise, a muscle-strengthening exercise or finishing stretch, and some extra suggestions – Bonus Burners – for when you feel like even more of a workout. Carry out the aerobic or anaerobic exercise first for the set amount of time, followed by the Bonus Burner if you feel like it. Then finish with the muscle-strengthener for the set number of repetitions.
▶ The programme makes use of the following equipment: stop watch, step bench, football, skipping rope, music, weights – both light medium and heavy (the weight will depend on your body frame to a certain extent, but should be approximately 1.5kg (3lb) to 5kg (11lb) – exercise trampoline and a Swiss ball (or large, air-filled ball).
▶ Try to do the routine every day. The 24 hours between bouts of exercise is sufficient to allow your muscles to recover. (You could follow the programme over 2 months if you would prefer to start slowly, by exercising every other day.)
▶ Keep at it. Don't let the fact that you have missed one day (or even two or three) put you off.
▶ Always warm-up and cool-down (see pages 48–51) to ensure you begin and end your programme safely.
▶ Always wear several layers of clothing so that the body warms up quickly. Strip off as you go flat out, then pile the layers back on to keep the heat in as you stretch out at the end.
▶ For exercise to work best it must be vigorous and prolonged! Don't worry if

Caution

Take care when exercising, as obviously all activity carries a risk.

▶ Before starting any exercise plan check that your doctor is happy for you to undertake a programme of self-supervised exercise.

▶ If you have not exercised in a long while, then take things very slowly and build up the level gradually.

▶ Be guided by how you feel when exercising. If you feel shattered the day after your activity, tone it down until the feeling you get the following day is one of healthy wellbeing.

this seems frightening now – after a few days of this programme you will become enthusiastic, seeking the challenge of doing more not less!

▶ Don't train if you get flu or a heavy cold (see below). If you have an injury or develop one during training, seek professional advice as to whether you can work around it and carry on.

Keeping going – 30 days and beyond

Refer to these guidelines to help you stick to your fitness programme.

If you feel ill
There is conflicting advice as to whether one should exercise when feeling ill. Listen to your body. If you have a really heavy cold or flu you won't feel like exercising – so don't do it. Give your body a few days to fight the infection and see how you feel. As we get older, bugs and viruses can take longer to get over so give yourself time to recover. Although it is important to keep going with your programme – a few rest days here or there will not lose your results.

Once you start to feel better, but still sluggish, then try a gentle session. Perhaps do just the warming up and cooling down part of the programme. Some gentle exercise will help get you back on the road to full health. The most important advice here is listen to your body and restart when it feels right.

If you feel stiff
Stiffness usually occurs when the body does something it is not used to, so you may feel stiff in the early stages of your exercise programme. One of the best ways to get rid of stiffness is to repeat the routine that made you stiff in the first place, although this can be quite painful as you do it. If the stiffness is really bad, give yourself 48 hours rest and some hot showers and aspirin.

If you feel fed up
We all feel demotivated from time to time. It's natural. It may be something going on outside your exercise life, which is intruding. Try to make time for the exercise, as at a stressful time you need it more than ever. If you really can't get going one day, let it go. Don't beat yourself up over it or use it as a reason to give up. Tell yourself that tomorrow is another chance to feel healthy.

If you feel over-enthusiastic
Your programme is going really well but you're eager for results. Perhaps you think you should double up on some of the routines or do it day and night? Don't be tempted to overdo things. Try to keep your enthusiasm for long-term application not for short-term intensity. Overdoing it could cause stiffness, which will put you off, or worse still, injury, which would really set you back. Take it easy and take your time.

If you feel hungover
Two major side effects of over-imbibing are tiredness and dehydration. So drink plenty and exercise anyway. You'll feel lousy, but it will get the blood flowing, carrying the waste products through your system, thus helping you feel on top of the hangover quicker. It may also remind you not to do it again in a hurry!

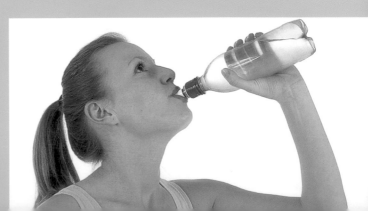

Warming up

Warming up is a must every time that you exercise. A warm-up is exactly what it says – a way of creating heat in the body. As you move, you build up heat in the muscles, making them more pliable and less prone to tearing or pulling. A warm-up should also involve mobilization of the joints, so that the warmed synovial fluid between the surfaces gives smooth movements. The warm-up phase is also a good time to practise with care any of the moves you might later do at speed. This should take you 10–15 minutes.

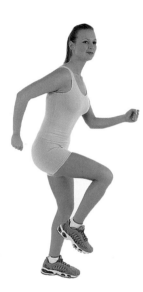

Floor march

1 March for five to ten minutes – to music if this helps – until you feel warmth radiating through your body. Swing your arms and lift your knees progressively higher and you should feel your breathing begin to increase. Try to step through your whole foot, i.e. roll from the toe through the ball of the foot to the heel as you step. This will mobilize the joints of the feet, ready for jumping and leaping later.

Body twist

1 Stand with your legs apart. Swing your arms out and around the body, to one side then the other.

2 Let the movement pull the upper half of the body around with it, so that you start to twist. Let the head and shoulders naturally follow the arms as they pull you around to each side. Do not allow the twist to go below the hips or you may be in danger of twisting your knees. As you twist you are warming up the torso and mobilizing the waist and the spine. Perform five to ten twists.

Side bends

1 As with the body twist exercise, you are mobilizing and warming up the torso, but adding a stretch. Stand with your feet hip-width apart. Reach with one arm down the side of your body towards your knee, letting the body stretch over to this side.

2 Return to upright, thinking of contracting the muscles on the other side of the torso to bring you up.

3 Repeat on the other side. Stretch 10–12 reaches to each side, keeping the movement flowing.

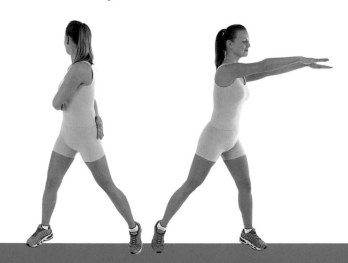

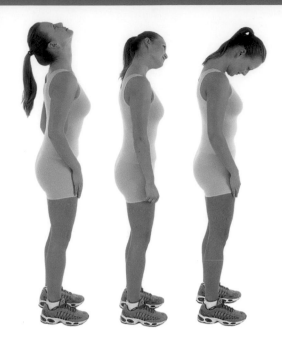

Pliés

1 Pliés are one of the best exercises for warming up the hips and legs. Stand with your legs more than hip-width apart, your feet slightly turned out, in a wide 'second position'. As you bend your knees, drop your bottom directly between your hips – do not stick it out behind you. Bend your knees so they align exactly over the toes.

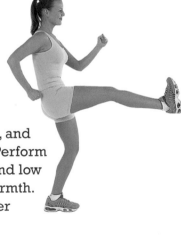

2 Bend your knees until they are at right angles and then slowly straighten again.

3 Perform 10–12 fluid repetitions.

Shoulder and head rolls

1 To warm up your neck area, first move your shoulders in several large circles. Lift them towards your ears and 'roll' them back behind you, then move them the other way. This warms up the shoulder area and builds heat in the neck.

2 Now begin to move your head. Drop it towards the floor then lift it to look at the ceiling. Note, there is a nerve in the back of the neck that is easily trapped, so don't drop your head backwards, simply tilt the head gently upwards in a controlled manner. Repeat four or five times.

3 Now look around over your right shoulder as far as you can, keeping your torso facing forward, then turn to look over your left shoulder. Repeat four to five times.

Dynamic stretch kicks

1 These kicks warm the leg muscles and briefly stretch the hamstrings. Stand with one foot in front of the other with your weight balanced.

2 Swing your back leg forward, slightly bent, and straighten it into a kick. Perform several kicks quite fast and low to build a rhythm and warmth. Then repeat with the other leg.

Jogging on the spot

1 You are now warmed up enough to move on to your main workout. Finish with some light jogging on the spot to get your breathing going and warm your feet and ankles.

Cooling down and stretching out

After any workout you must give your body time to cool down before you shower. Use these exercises to bring you back to reality after your fab workout. Note, these stretches can also be done before you work out to ready the muscles for action.

Marching on the spot – cooling down

1 March on the spot to give yourself a chance to catch your breath, or simply keep walking or stepping gently, before you sit down. This will allow your heart a gradual recovery and the muscles to stop contracting slowly. Once you feel the heat start to leave your body slightly, you can begin to stretch the muscles you have used. Stretching returns the contracted muscles to their original length, and helps prevent stiffness and promote flexibility.

Hamstring stretch

1 Start by stretching out your leg muscles. Lie on the floor and lift one leg up till you can catch hold of it with your hands. Hold the leg as straight as you can bear it.

2 Now gently rotate your ankle first one way and then the other. Then gently pull in the leg a little farther if you can. Hold and release.

3 Repeat with the other leg.

Calf stretch

1 Stand in a lunge position with one leg stretched behind you. Bend the front knee to lean forward, while pressing the back heel down.

2 Hold this position for 10–12 seconds, feeling a stretch in the calf muscle (the back of the lower leg). It is prone to cramp, so stretch it regularly. Change legs and repeat.

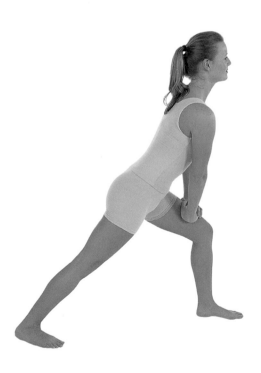

Quad stretch

1 Stand on one leg with a hand on the wall to balance you. Grasp the other foot with the other hand.

2 Press the heel of the foot towards your bottom, while pressing your hips forward and pulling in on your abdominals. Hold for 10–12 seconds to stretch the quadriceps muscle (the front of the thigh). Repeat on the other leg.

All-over lean

1 Hold the back of a sturdy chair and walk your legs away until your body is at right angles.

2 Try to relax into and hold this position for 10–12 seconds – keeping the abdominal muscles working for some support. You will

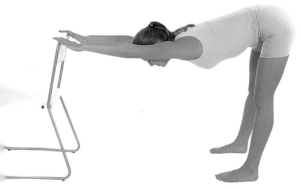

feel a stretch in the shoulders and backs of your legs, and should feel a pleasant flexing of the lower back (the lumbar spine area). Walk yourself back to standing.

Swing out

1 Well done! You have completed your workout and stretched your body. Breathing deeply, gently swing and shake your arms around the body, up above your head and down towards your feet – bending your knees.

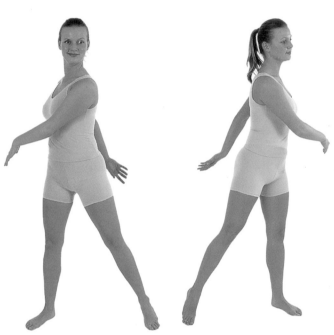

Caution

The theory behind cooling down is that you should never stop vigorous exercise suddenly as the blood is pumping strongly and could cause a blockage. The circulation needs time to return to a more normal pace. The body also needs time to cool down and for the muscles to be released from their strong contractions. So always bring your heart rate down gradually with slower exercise before you stop moving completely.

day 1

DON'T FORGET
► To warm up before (see pages 48–49)
► To cool down after (see pages 50–51)

Aerobic Exercise: Walking

Find somewhere you can walk without too much to stop you, like a park or even a shopping centre. Set your watch and keep going for 15 minutes.

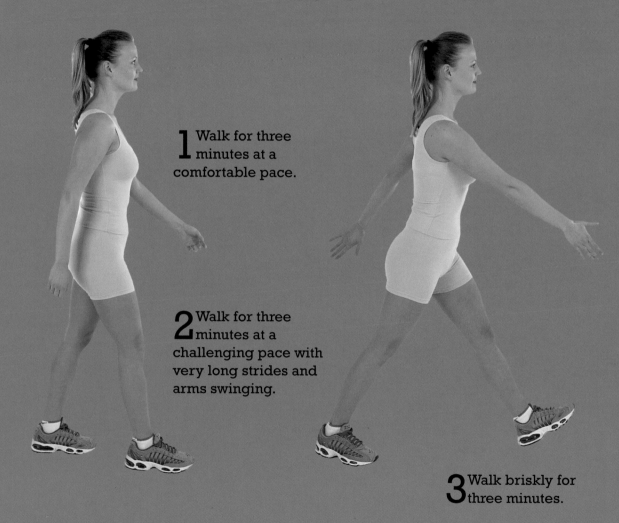

1 Walk for three minutes at a comfortable pace.

2 Walk for three minutes at a challenging pace with very long strides and arms swinging.

3 Walk briskly for three minutes.

Bonus Burner

► Walk so fast that you break into a run. Repeat three times.

► Count how many strides you take to cover a length of the park or mall. Lengthen your stride and reduce the number of steps you take.

► Repeat the walking sequence five times.

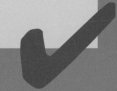

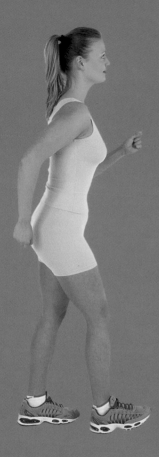

Technique Points

▶ When you are walking for fitness you should be breathing fairly heavily. Don't dawdle – as you might when on a shopping trip – but step out purposefully.

Muscle Stengthener:
All fours press-up *repeat ten times*

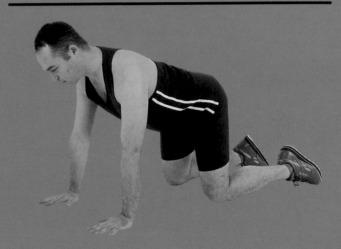

4 Walk for three minutes with shortened strides (smaller steps than you would normally take).

5 Walk for two minutes fast, followed by one minute at a comfortable pace.

6 Walk backwards, or raise your knees to your chest as you walk.

1 Get on to your hands and knees and lean forward to put some weight on your hands. Keep your neck in line with your spine at all times.

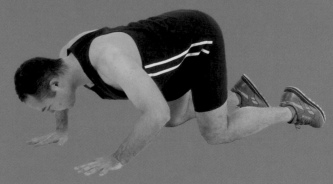

2 Now bend your arms and touch your nose to the floor, then straighten your arms, keeping your tummy tight.

53

day 2

DON'T FORGET
► To warm up before (see pages 48–49)
► To cool down after (see pages 50–51)

Aerobic Exercise: Step routine

Today you are taking your walking to a new level; up and down! Stepping onto a bench will increase the intensity of your workout and adds variation. Set your watch and keep going for 20 minutes.

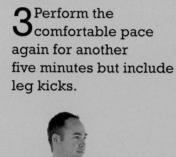

3 Perform the comfortable pace again for another five minutes but include leg kicks.

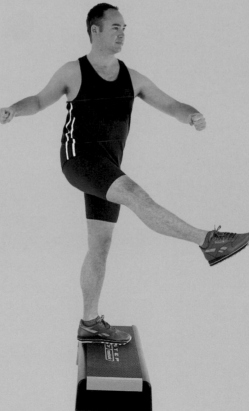

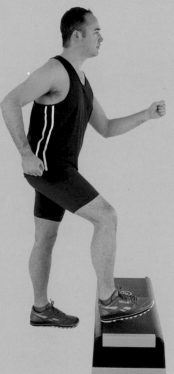

4 Do another five minutes of increased pace with added arm movements and alternate between leg kicks and knee lifts.

1 Step up and down on to a step bench for five minutes at a comfortable pace.

2 Increase the pace for another five minutes.

Technique Points

► Ensure your feet are always fully on the step bench. Keep your knees bent slightly when on top of the step and keep your chest lifted.

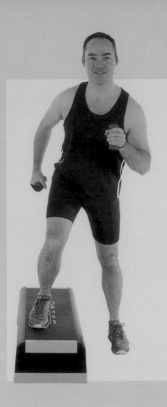

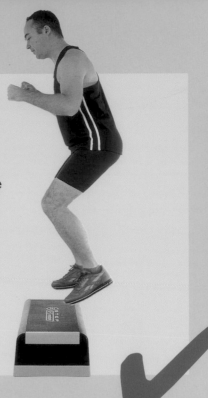

Bonus Burner

▶ Carry or wear light wrist weights to add resistance.

▶ For some of the time, jump with both feet together on to the step rather than stepping up.

Muscle Strengthener: Stomach curl-ups *repeat 30 times*

1 Lie on your back and cross your ankles together in the air.

2 With your hands supporting your head, curl up your torso so that your elbows reach towards your knees.

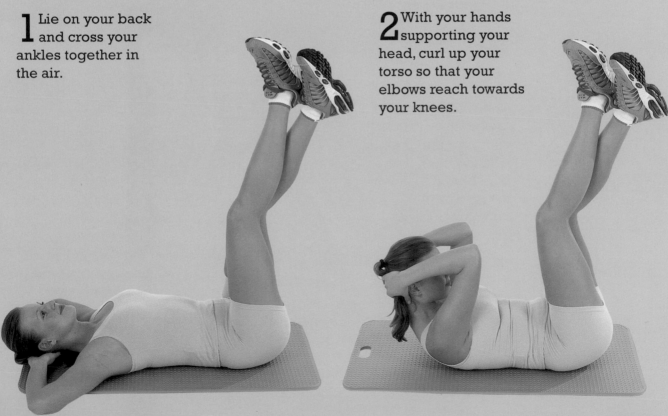

55

day 3

DON'T FORGET
▶ To warm up before (see pages 48–49)
▶ To cool down after (see pages 50–51)

Aerobic Exercise: Shadow boxing

Start by jogging from one foot to the other then add in some of the punches and moves below in three-minute rounds. Have a one-minute breather between rounds and do 20 stomach curl-ups (see Day 2, page 55). Keep going for 20 minutes

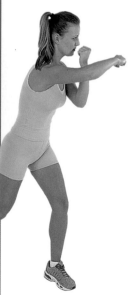

Jab

1 Start with both hands up near your face for protection.

2 Now extend one arm sharply and recoil it to perform the jab. You are aiming for your phantom partner's jaw!

Uppercut

1 The uppercut punch comes from low down, so bend your knees and swing the weight of your whole body upwards as you aim to punch up underneath your phantom partner's ribcage!

Hook

1 The hook punch comes around the side. Bring your arm around in a semicircle with your arm parallel with the floor. This punch would land on the side of your opponent's head!

Punch dodging

1 With your feet wide apart, use your whole torso and bend your legs to get low as the imaginary punches come at your head.

2 Bob up and bob back down again as fast as you can.

Bonus Burner

▶ During the break between rounds, do burpees (see below) instead of stomach curl-ups after every other round.

▶ Aim to keep bouncing at all times during each round, with no standing still on your feet at any stage.

Technique Points

▶ Stand at all times in a pyramid position in relation to the object of your punches. (This makes you a smaller target in real boxing.)

▶ Keep your hands up as though to guard your face at all times when not in use.

▶ Use some upbeat music.

Muscle Strengthener: Burpees *repeat 20 times*

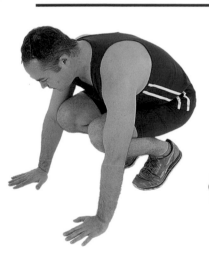
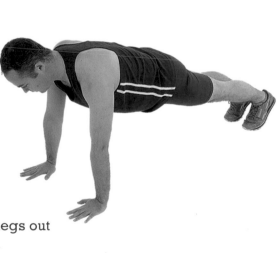
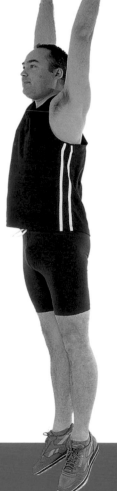

1 Start in a low squat position.

2 Shoot your legs out behind you.

3 Then shoot them back in again and push with your leg muscles to leap upwards into the air – the more of a rhythm you get going, the easier the exercise will become!

day 4

DON'T FORGET
▶ To warm up before (see pages 48–49)
▶ To cool down after (see pages 50–51)

Aerobic Exercise: Exercise trampoline

Aim to perform up to 20 minutes of continuous jogging
and leaping on the exercise trampoline by alternating between the
moves suggested below.

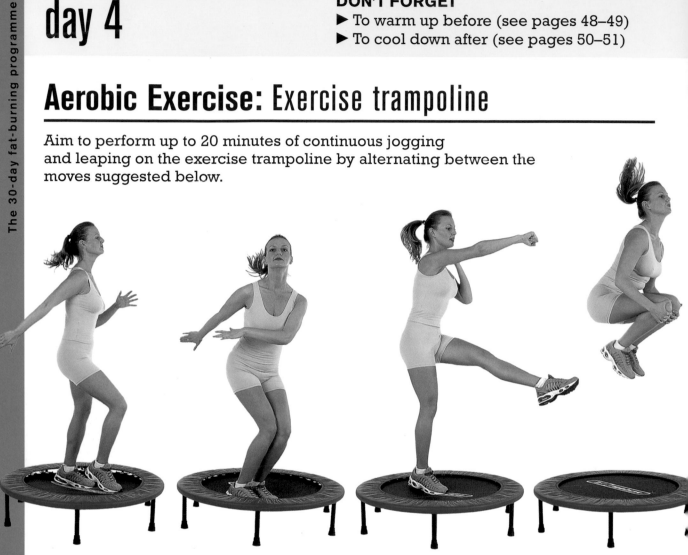

1 Start by walking while pressing your heels deep into the bed of the trampoline.

2 Build up to real jogging with knees high and add in an occasional jump with a twist as you land.

3 Utilize different movements such as one-knee-to-chest hops, twisting from side to side, and front leg kicks. Throw in some shadow boxing moves learned in Day 3 (see page 56).

4 Bend your knees to push off into a high jump with both legs. Try to tuck your knees right up towards your chest, keeping the chest lifted, then extend your legs again to land on your feet.

Bonus Burner

▶ Include some step lunges (see Day 13, page 76) with one foot off the exercise trampoline, and skip from one side of the trampoline to the other.

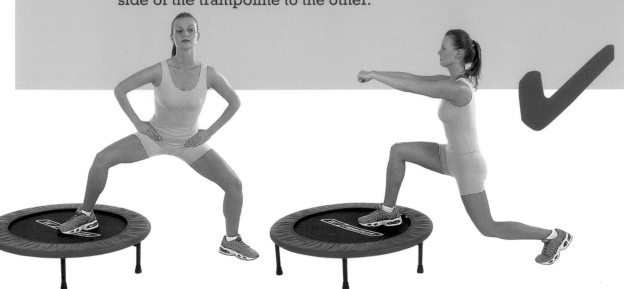

Muscle Strengthener:
Ab swapsees *repeat 20 times*

Technique Points

▶ When using the trampoline it is important to make sure you press your heels all the way down on each landing (otherwise your calves will ache). Keep the knees slightly bent and pull in on your stomach area and pelvic floor for support.

1 Lie on your back on the trampoline and place your hands on the edge of the frame. Rest your head but lift your legs, keeping one bent and the other straight.

2 Swap the legs immediately, straightening the bent leg and bending the other one. You will feel this exercise in your stomach.

day 5

DON'T FORGET
▶ To warm up before (see pages 48–49)
▶ To cool down after (see pages 50–51)

Anaerobic Exercise: Heavy weights workout

Today you are using weights to build muscle. This will use up even more calories. This should take approximately 30 minutes.

1 March up and down for five minutes, lifting your knees as high as you can while holding a 5kg (12lb) dumbbell in front of you.

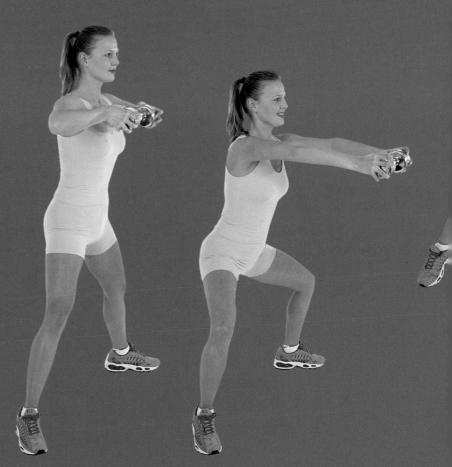

2 Standing with your legs apart, bend and straighten your legs as you press the dumbbell out in front of you and pull it back in again. Repeat this 25 times.

3 March on the spot, lifting the dumbbell up and down again.

Bonus Burner

▶ Try this with progressively heavier weights until you can only manage ten repetitions of each exercise.

Muscle Strengthener:
Leg extension *repeat ten times on each leg*

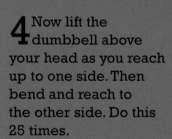

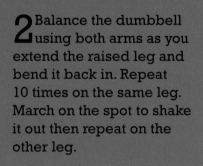

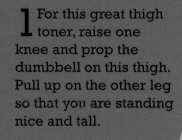

1 For this great thigh toner, raise one knee and prop the dumbbell on this thigh. Pull up on the other leg so that you are standing nice and tall.

4 Now lift the dumbbell above your head as you reach up to one side. Then bend and reach to the other side. Do this 25 times.

5 March on the spot, lifting the dumbbell up and down, as before.

6 March on the spot and then repeat the whole sequence three times. This should keep you going for 30 minutes.

2 Balance the dumbbell using both arms as you extend the raised leg and bend it back in. Repeat 10 times on the same leg. March on the spot to shake it out then repeat on the other leg.

Technique Points

▶ Throughout these exercises where you are lifting something heavy, remember to pull in on your abdominals and pelvic floor muscles. As you tighten the abdominals they will support your torso and maintain your posture to keep the body safe as you lift.

day 6

DON'T FORGET
► To warm up before (see pages 48–49)
► To cool down after (see pages 50–51)

Anaerobic Exercise: Circuit-type session

A circuit gives you a range of different exercises to try while keeping your heart rate raised. Aim to keep moving for 20 minutes.

What is an Activity Station? An activity station is just that. You should perform a chosen activity for a set amount of time before moving on to the next station. All the stations together will make one circuit.

1 Set five different activity stations. Perform at each station for one minute and jog on the spot to recover between each station for 30 seconds.

● **Station 1:** Rope skipping (see Day 15, page 80)

● **Station 2:** Shadow boxing (see Day 3, page 56)

● **Station 3:** Burpees (see Day 3, page 57)

● **Station 4:** Stepping (see Day 2, page 54)

● **Station 5:** Rebounding (see Day 4, page 58)

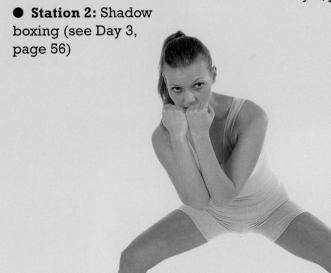

2 Repeat the circuit of all five stations four times.

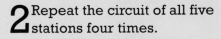

Bonus Burner

▶ Do each station for up to two minutes at a time, but repeat the circuit three times.

▶ Aim to perform more rope skipping at Station 1 and burpees at Station 3.

▶ Add another station or two of your choice.

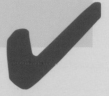

Technique Points

▶ If you find you can't keep a rhythm going while using the skipping rope then chuck it aside and do the movements without the rope.

Muscle Strengthener: Tension hold

1 Start on all fours, then lift the knees to assume the position illustrated. Squeeze your bottom tight and pull up the abdominals to maintain the plank position. Keep your neck in line with your spine.

2 Keep breathing while you hold this position for 30 seconds. Rest then repeat once more, or twice if you can. This exercise will tone the shoulders, abdominals, back and legs.

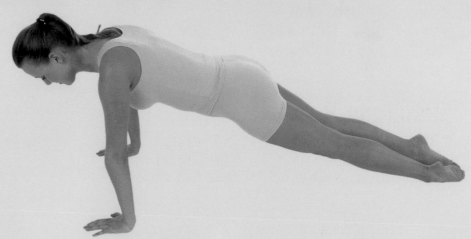

day 7

DON'T FORGET
▶ To warm up before (see pages 48–49)
▶ To cool down after (see pages 50–51)

Aerobic Exercise: Running

Choose your pace – comfortable, brisk or fast – according to your fitness level and keep moving for 15 minutes.

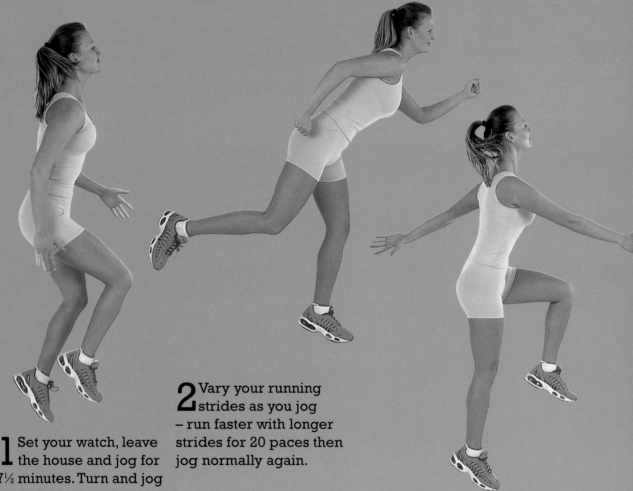

1 Set your watch, leave the house and jog for 7½ minutes. Turn and jog back the way you came.

2 Vary your running strides as you jog – run faster with longer strides for 20 paces then jog normally again.

3 Pick your knees right up and jog vertically for 20 paces then jog normally again.

Technique Points

▶ Run slowly to begin with so that you can keep going. Place your heels down first and roll through the foot. Breathe evenly, trying to get into a rhythm.

Bonus Burner

▶ After five minutes, sprint for one minute. Repeat three times.

▶ Increase the above sprint time to 90 seconds.

▶ Increase the running time to 10–15 minutes on the way out, and the same on the way back for a 20–30 minute run in total when you feel fitter.

Muscle Strengthener:
Shoulder stand practice *repeat five times*

1 Lie on your back on the floor. Bend your knees to help you roll your back off the floor. If you can only get your hips up this is fine. Use your hands to support your hips.

2 If you can, roll your back right off the floor into a shoulder stand, using your hands for support. Hold for several seconds, roll down and rest. Repeat four more times.

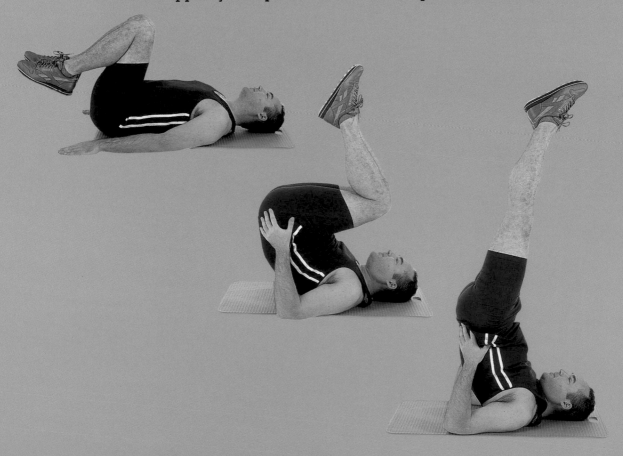

day 8

DON'T FORGET
► To warm up before (see pages 48–49)
► To cool down after (see pages 50–51)

Aerobic Exercise: Pyramid circuit training

Using the pyramid method as explained in the box below, this aerobic circuit should take 25–30 minutes if performed twice. At each station perform the exercise for just 30 seconds. Between each level perform an exercise 'break': run 10 metres (10 yards), turn and run back.

How does the pyramid method work?

The pyramid method is a great way to work out. It involves choosing six activities, each of which you perform at a different station, either for a set number of repetitions or for a given time.

As illustrated below, you start the session at the top of the pyramid with station 1, followed by an exercise break of light exercise. Then you move down to the next level, where you perform the activities at stations 1 and 2 before repeating the break, and so on down the pyramid. This type of circuit allows you to know precisely what you have done. By the end of the session you will surprise yourself at how many repetitions you have done in total.

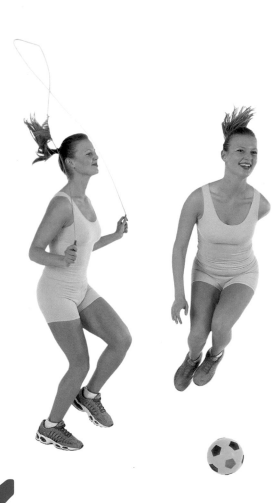

```
                    1
              EXERCISE BREAK
               1     2
            EXERCISE BREAK
            1     2     3
         EXERCISE BREAK
         1     2     3     4
      EXERCISE BREAK
      1     2     3     4     5
   EXERCISE BREAK
   1     2     3     4     5     6
```

● **Station 1: Rope skipping** (see Day 15, page 80)

● **Station 2: Jumping side to side** over a ball (see Day 16, page 82)

● **Station 3: Hopping on the spot**, first with one leg then with the other

● **Station 4: Bounding**: jogging with large paces, pushing hard off each foot (see Day 13, page 76)

● **Station 5: Stepping on to a step** bench then stepping back down (see Day 2, page 54)

● **Station 6: Jumping with two feet** on to a step bench and stepping back down (see Day 2, page 55)

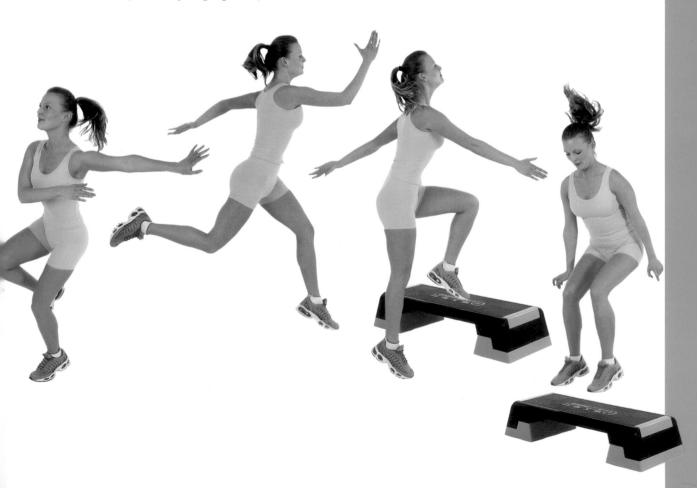

day 9

DON'T FORGET
► To warm up before (see pages 48–49)
► To cool down after (see pages 50–51)

Aerobic Exercise: Light weights workout

Today you are using light weights (1–1½lb) to increase the intensity of your aerobics. Using the weights, perform each of the exercises suggested here consecutively 20 times – in either single or double time. Keep your feet moving all the time where possible – either by marching or stepping from side to side – while performing the moves. Between each exercise step from side-to-side swinging your arms. This should keep you moving for 25 minutes.

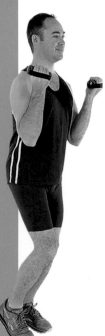

Bicep curls

1 Start by holding the weights by your sides. Carefully bend your arms, turning the weights inwards as you bend.

2 Hold then release your arms down slowly – this works the muscles along the front of your arms.

Pec decs

1 Hold your arms bent and out to the side at right angles.

2 Press the elbows forward so that you bring them together in front of your chest.

3 Hold and open again to repeat. This will work the pectoral muscles on the chest.

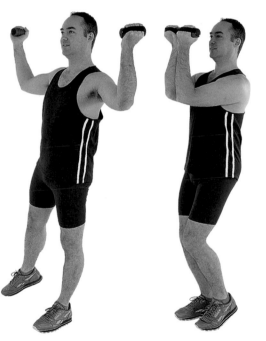

Tricep kick-back

1 Step backwards while lifting your elbows up into the air behind you and then press the dumbbells upwards to straighten the arms. You will feel the muscle in the back of each arm working as you straighten it.

2 Bend your arms back down as you step forward.

Shoulder press

1 Stand with your knees slightly bent, feet hip-width apart and ribcage and chest lifted. With a weight in each hand bend your arms to your shoulders.

2 Press the weights directly up to the ceiling and lower slowly. Eight repetitions will work your shoulder muscles (the deltoids).

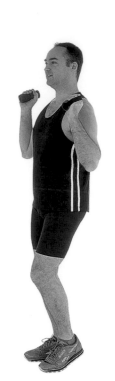
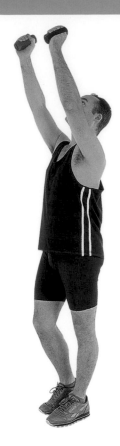

Muscle Strengthener:
Weighted exercises

1 Perform some of the above exercises more slowly with heavier weights. Use a 5–10kg (1–2lb) dumbbell if you can and use a slow count of four as you lift and then lower the weight.

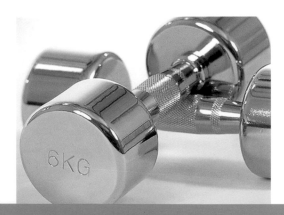

Bonus Burner

▶ Increase the repetitions.

▶ Take a shorter break between sets.

▶ Try adding some other exercises with weights, such as a one-arm row (see Day 18, page 86) and lateral raises (see Day 21, page 92).

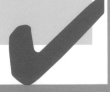

day 10

DON'T FORGET
► To warm up before (see pages 48–49)
► To cool down after (see pages 50–51)

Aerobic Exercise: Stairs workout

Use your stairs at home or some steps in a local park to do 20 minutes of cardiovascular work.

1 Run up and down the stairs three times to get warm.

2 Run up one step and back down. Run up two steps and back down, then up and down three steps and so on, until you have been all the way up and down.

3 Then go up and down the stairs two at a time.

Technique Points
► Watch that your knees are in line with your toes as you step upwards. On the way down pull up on the abdominals to support your back and step through the toes to the heel to protect your knees, whilst stepping down at a slant (see picture below).

4 When you get to the top of the stairs perform five small feet-together jumps.

5 Finish with three trips up and down the stairs.

Bonus Burner
► Try going up the stairs three at a time, coming back down the normal way.

► Use some lightweights while you do this workout.

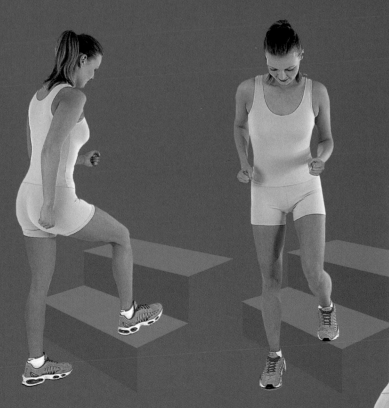

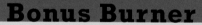

Muscle Strengthener:
Squat thrusts with bunny jump *repeat 20 times*

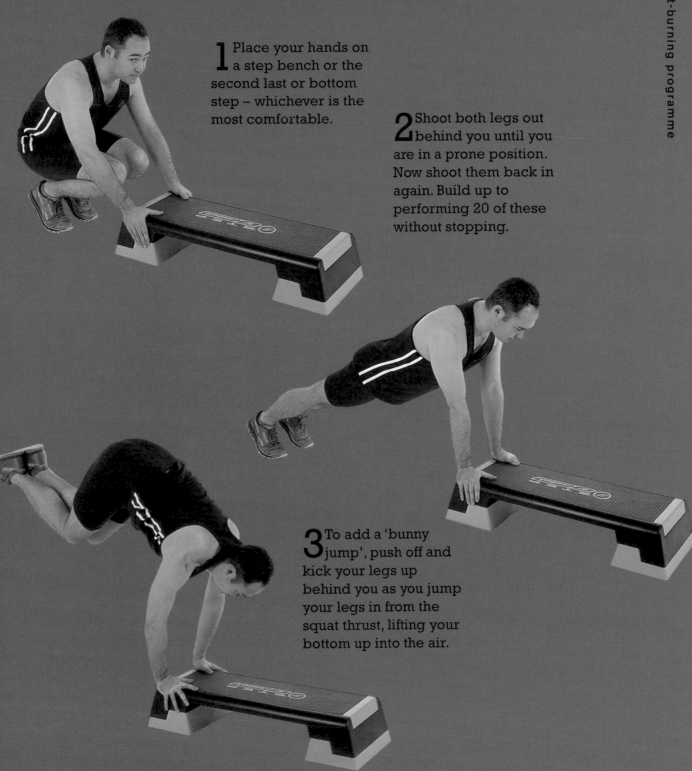

1 Place your hands on a step bench or the second last or bottom step – whichever is the most comfortable.

2 Shoot both legs out behind you until you are in a prone position. Now shoot them back in again. Build up to performing 20 of these without stopping.

3 To add a 'bunny jump', push off and kick your legs up behind you as you jump your legs in from the squat thrust, lifting your bottom up into the air.

day 11

DON'T FORGET
► To warm up before (see pages 48–49)
► To cool down after (see pages 50–51)

Aerobic Exercise: Pyramid circuit with Swiss ball

This is the same pyramid principle as Day 8 (see pages 66–67), but the exercises here are using the versatile Swiss ball. At each station perform 10 complete repetitions of the exercise. Between each level perform a 1-minute exercise 'break': jog for 1 minute while holding and pumping the Swiss Ball above your head.

● **Station 1: Pelvic tilts on ball**

1 Sit comfortably on the ball, making sure you are pulling up through the spine and sitting tall.

2 Using your stomach muscles, gently move your hips from side to side to roll the ball beneath you, tilting it first one way then the other.

● **Station 2: Jumping jacks**

1 Hold the Swiss ball in front of you and jump up, landing with feet wide apart.

2 Bend the knees gently as you land. Repeat in rhythm.

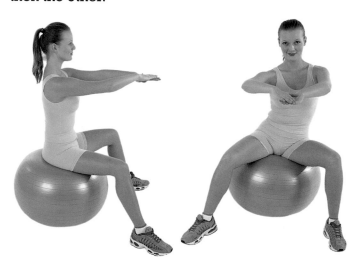

● **Station 3: Back arches**

1 Lie over the Swiss ball with your head resting forward and your hands behind your head.

2 Now lift your head and shoulders off the ball, arching backwards and then lower them again. This works the erector spinae muscles that run along either side of your spine.

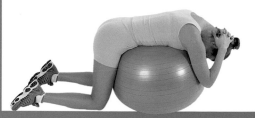

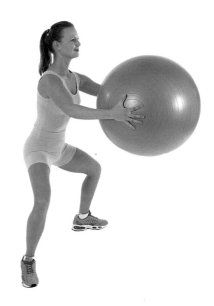

● Station 4:
Press-ups on ball

1 Lie on top of the ball, face down, and take your weight on to your hands.

2 Slowly walk your hands out so that the ball rolls down towards your knees. Use your upper legs to control it as you bend and straighten your arms in a press-up (see Day 15, page 80).

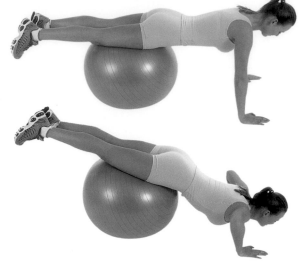

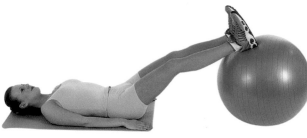

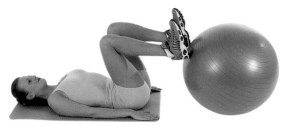

● Station 5: Hamstring curls

1 Lie on your back and drape your legs over the ball.

2 Flex your feet and use your heels to inch the ball towards you, bending your knees. You will feel your hamstrings working.

3 Gently roll out the ball until your legs are straight again.

● Station 6: Swiss ball curl-ups

1 Lie backwards over the ball and plant your feet firmly on the ground and your hands behind your head.

2 Perform a curl-up. These curl-ups are tougher than doing the same on the floor (see Day 2, page 55), because you are coming up from an incline position.

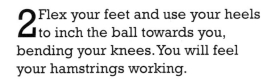

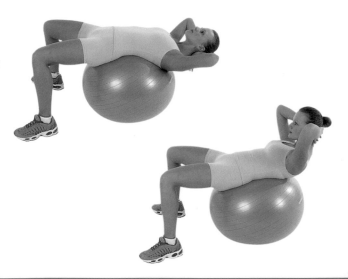

73

day 12

DON'T FORGET
► To warm up before (see pages 48–49)
► To cool down after (see pages 50–51)

Aerobic Exercise: Exercise trampoline 2

You are on the hop again today, this time for 30 minutes. Use the moves from Day 4 (page 58) but add some more adventurous feet-together jumps and turns and torso twists. Try cat jumps, W-jumps or star jumps to really get your breathing going.

Cat jumps

1 Tuck your feet up behind you as you spring into the air and arch your back slightly, reaching one arm behind you towards your feet.

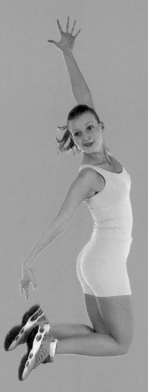

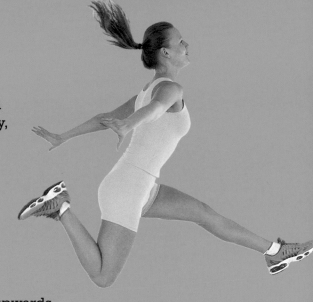

W-jumps

1 Spring upwards, extending one leg forward and bending the other back. Fling both arms straight behind you.

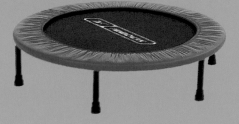

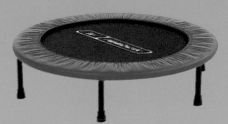

Bonus Burner

► Try some quarter-, half- and full turns on your trampoline.

Star jumps

1 Take off with both feet and, as you push upwards, shoot both your legs and arms out to the side in a star position.

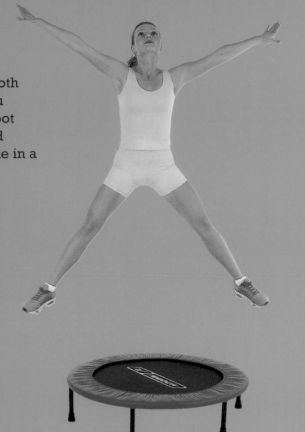

Technique Points

▶ Make sure you jump from the middle of the trampoline and try to land there. Start with low jumps and build up to higher leaps as you gain more confidence.

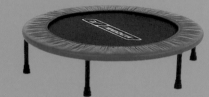

Muscle Strengthener:
Buttockblaster *repeat 20 times on each leg*

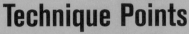

1 This exercise will tone and strengthen the buttocks. Tip your trampoline on its side and hold on to two of its legs for balance.

2 Now lean forward and lift one leg behind you. Keep the leg straight and lift it, hold for one second then lower it.

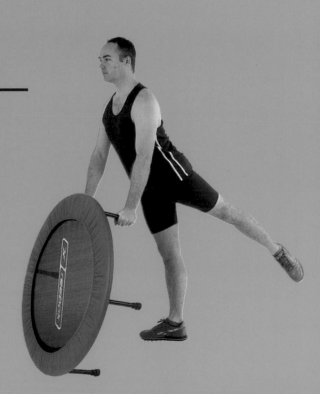

day 13

DON'T FORGET
▶ To warm up before (see pages 48–49)
▶ To cool down after (see pages 50–51)

Anaerobic Exercise: Plyometrics

Plyometric exercises are high intensity moves designed to boost calorie burning. Use the park so that you have plenty of room to move. Warm up by walking briskly or jogging for five minutes. Jog one length of the park and then try each of the following moves as you come back again. Keep going for 20 minutes.

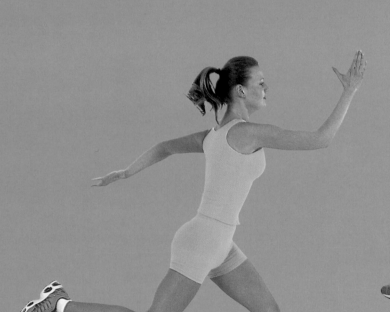

Bounding

1 Start by jogging with large paces.

2 As you jog, push off each foot as much as you can so that you are spending longer in the air between each step. The actual pacing will be slower but you will use more energy as you push off the ground.

Step lunges

1 Stand on the spot and step in front of you into a lunge position. Both legs should be bent with your weight evenly distributed between them.

2 Push forward with your back leg to step into another lunge in front.

3 Keep alternating as you step right across the park.

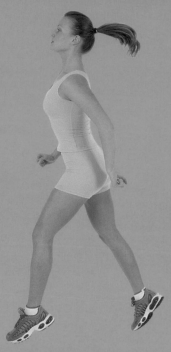

Technique Points

▶ It is important when doing any kind of jump that you check the alignment of your knees. As they bend, ensure that your heels are pressed down and that your knees don't push beyond your toes.

Muscle Strengthener:
Tricep dips *repeat 40 times*

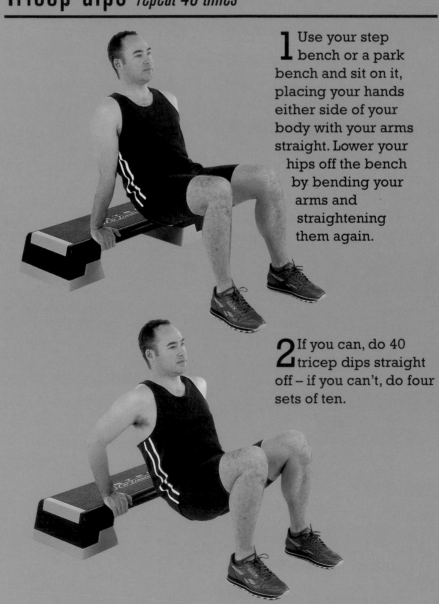

Lunge jumps

1 Now that you have practised the lunge position (see left), assume the position but this time push upwards from this position into a jump.

2 Land back down into the lunge, going through the feet and bending the knees so that there is no jarring on the legs.

3 Change legs and repeat.

Change leg lunge jumps

1 As you leap upwards from your lunge jump, change your legs while in the air so that you land with your other foot in front.

1 Use your step bench or a park bench and sit on it, placing your hands either side of your body with your arms straight. Lower your hips off the bench by bending your arms and straightening them again.

2 If you can, do 40 tricep dips straight off – if you can't, do four sets of ten.

77

day 14

DON'T FORGET
▶ To warm up before (see pages 48–49)
▶ To cool down after (see pages 50–51)

Aerobic Exercise: Shadow boxing 2

Use the punches and techniques you learned on Day 3 (page 56), as well as the moves shown below. Complete the moves in 3-minute rounds, beginning with the 'Ali shuffle'. Add a lot more aggression: think of someone (or something!) you really dislike and go for it! Aim for eight rounds of three minutes each.

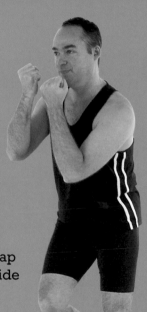

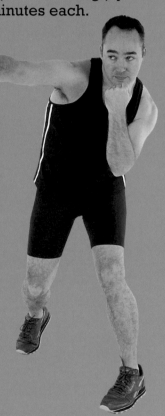

Power punch

1 This follows on from the jab (see Day 3, page 56). As you recoil from the jab with one hand, swing the other arm across the body and punch with full force.

2 Swivel on the ball of your foot to swerve, so the full force of your body is behind the punch.

Ali shuffle

1 Jog and swap feet from side to side as you practise your punches.

2 Imagine you have an opponent and really try to increase the intensity and sharpness of your punches.

Bonus Burner

▶ Between rounds, do some squat thrusts (see Day 10, page 71, but without the step) or some change leg lunge jumps (see Day 13, page 77).

▶ Try to build up a sequence of moves to a count of eight and four each:
1. Jab, jab, powerpunch; speedball
2. Jab, uppercut, hook, hook; hook, duck, hook, duck

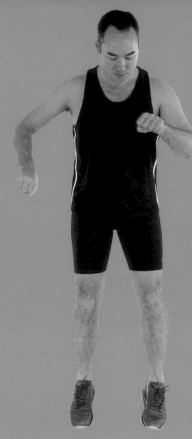

Shoe shine

1 Jog backwards, kicking your feet out in front of you (as you do when skipping) and skim your fist in the air in a horizontal circle as if you were buffing the shine on your trainers from above.

Speedball

1 Revolve your hands in a circle as fast and furiously as you can while aiming to hit the back of your hands on an imaginary punch bag.

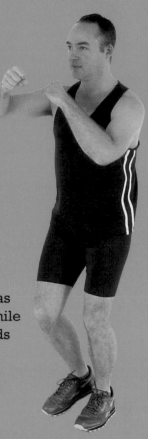

Muscle Strengthener: Back stretch *repeat 10–15 times*

1 To strengthen the back muscles that run either side of the spine, lie on your stomach and place your hands up by your ears.

2 Squeeze your buttocks as you lift your upper body and your lower legs as high as you can off the floor. Hold for five seconds and then release slowly breathing freely throughout

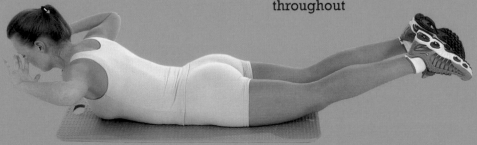

79

day 15

DON'T FORGET
► To warm up before (see pages 48–49)
► To cool down after (see pages 50–51)

Aerobic Exercise: Rope skipping

Skipping is hard, calorie-burning work, so take it steady and practise to keep the pace going at a reasonable level for 20–30 minutes.

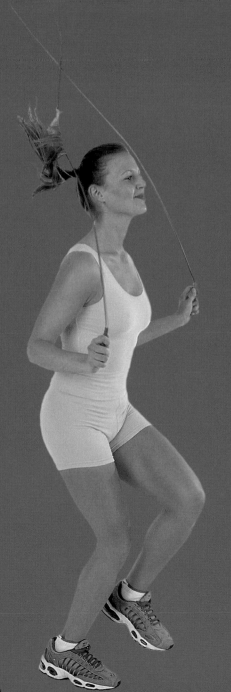

1 Skip for one minute at a comfortable pace.

2 Skip for one minute at a challenging pace.

3 Skip briskly for one minute.

4 Skip fast for 30 seconds, followed by 30 seconds at a comfortable pace. Ensure you keep this going for 20 minutes.

4 Skip backwards or raise your knees to your chest as you skip.

Bonus Burner

► Skip fast for 45 seconds, followed by only 15 seconds rest. Repeat three times.

► Test yourself to see how many skips you can achieve in one minute.

► Repeat the basic exercise five times instead of four.

Technique Points

▶ The key to consistent rope skipping is to keep your knees bent at all times and lift the feet only very slightly. Too many people try to leap over the rope. This is too exhausting and will only trip you up. Use your hamstrings to bend the knees and lift your feet up.

▶ Try flicking the skipping rope from your wrists – don't move your arms too much.

Muscle Strengthener: Full press-ups *repeat ten times*

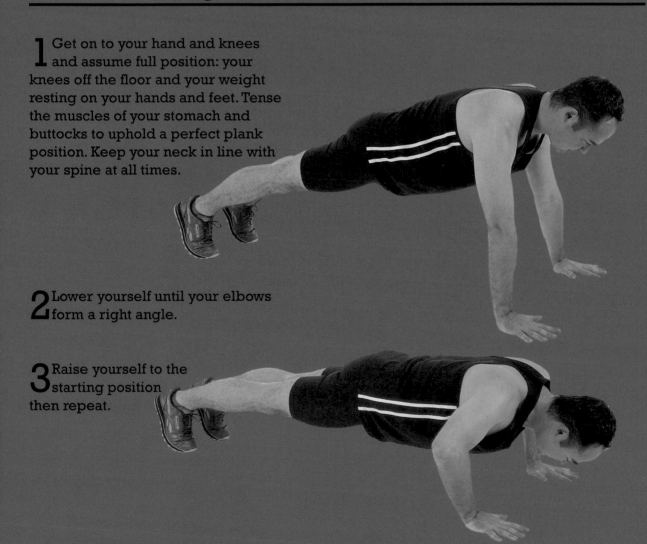

1 Get on to your hand and knees and assume full position: your knees off the floor and your weight resting on your hands and feet. Tense the muscles of your stomach and buttocks to uphold a perfect plank position. Keep your neck in line with your spine at all times.

2 Lower yourself until your elbows form a right angle.

3 Raise yourself to the starting position then repeat.

day 16

DON'T FORGET
► To warm up before (see pages 48–49)
► To cool down after (see pages 50–51)

Aerobic Exercise: Football circuit

Keep moving for 20 minutes using a football. This workout is best done outside but most of it could be done indoors, too, preferably with a soft ball!

1 Start jogging on the spot, holding on to the ball. As you jog, lift the ball up above your head and down again.

2 Lift your knees up high as you jog and swing the ball over your head from side to side. Keep this going for five minutes until you are really warm.

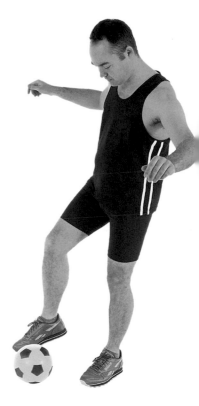

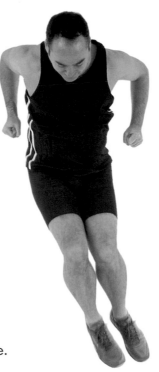

3 Now find yourself a length of park about 20m long and place the ball on the ground, halfway through your route. Sprint in and out and around the ball, sprinting from the start to the end position in between each round.

4 Place the ball on the ground and jump over the ball from side to side. Repeat for one minute.

5 Now 'dribble' the ball up and down the length of the park, keeping your feet in contact with the ball. Repeat for two minutes.

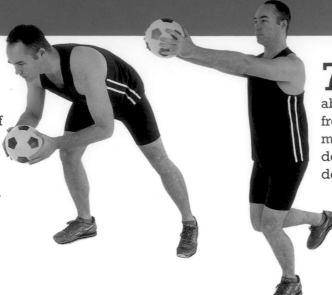

6 Pick up the ball, throw it ahead of you and sprint to catch it. Perform this five times in different directions.

7 Jog on the spot, pushing the ball up above your head or from side to side – in a mock cheer – to cool down. Bring the pace down to a walk.

Technique Points

▶ Get as low as you can each time you go to pick up the ball.

▶ When jumping, land through your feet and bend the knees.

Muscle Strengthener:
Reverse curls with ball *repeat ten times*

1 To tone the stomach, lie on the floor with your knees raised. Place the ball between your knees.

2 Now with bent legs pull your thighs in towards you and try to lift your hips off the floor. You are contracting your abdominals doing this and you will feel the work particularly in the lower part of your rectus abdominals.

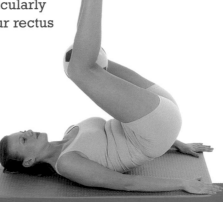

83

day 17

DON'T FORGET
▶ To warm up before (see pages 48–49)
▶ To cool down after (see pages 50–51)

Aerobic Exercise: Dance workout

Keep dancing for 20 minutes! This is your freeform workout and your chance to be creative. You can make this workout as hard as you want. Put on a piece of music that you love and really get moving!

1 Start off by jigging on the spot. Now think of every dance move you've ever known and start adding them in! Move your hips, swing your arms and leap and turn!

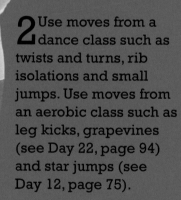

2 Use moves from a dance class such as twists and turns, rib isolations and small jumps. Use moves from an aerobic class such as leg kicks, grapevines (see Day 22, page 94) and star jumps (see Day 12, page 75).

Bonus Burner
▶ Repeat this workout on another day wearing wrist or ankle weights.

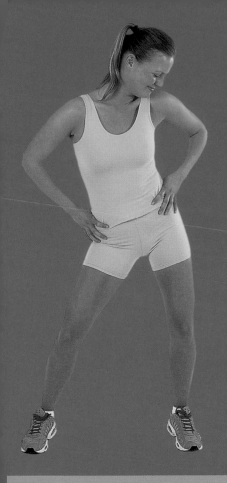

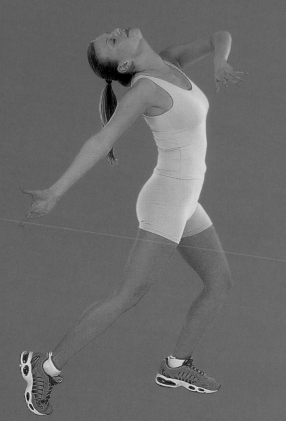

3 Use moves from the Lambada scene such as hip rotations, back leans and shoulder shimmies. Use moves from partner dances such as the waltz step, the Charleston and the cha-cha.

4 Use moves that you remember (or make up) from rock-and-roll movies and jive dances. Whatever you do, just keep moving, don't stop!

Technique Points

▶ The great thing about this workout is that it will challenge your brain's creativity as well as your body – using even more calories. Keep moving and make it a point of honour not to stop! You will probably find you will be more stiff afterwards from this workout than from any other. This is because you will have used muscles you didn't know (or had forgotten) you had.

Muscle Strengthener:
Ab cross curls *do five sets of 20*

1 Lie on your back and work your abdominals. Raise your feet just above the ground then draw up one knee and touch it with the opposite elbow.

2 Alternate your arms and legs and keep going until you have done five sets of 20 repetitions. Rest for only ten seconds in between sets.

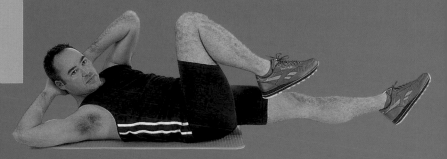

day 18

DON'T FORGET
► To warm up before (see pages 48–49)
► To cool down after (see pages 50–51)

Anaerobic Exercise: Upper body weights

This is another workout that is not about keeping going for 20 minutes or more. The focus here is on working the muscles hard – so hard you couldn't possibly keep it up for 20 minutes.

Tricep extensions

1 These will strengthen and tone the tricep muscle at the back of each arm. Stand with your feet hip-width apart and knees slightly bent. Pull in on your abdominals and lift your chest. Grasp a weight in one hand and hold it behind your head as shown. Use your other arm to support your position.

2 Now extend the arm so that the end of the dumbbell points towards the ceiling and then bend the arm again.

3 Do eight repetitions – which should be pretty challenging! If you need to, use your other arm to help.

One-arm row

1 This will strengthen and tone the upper back and the biceps on the upper arm. Step into a lunge and bend forward, with one hand holding the weight hanging towards the floor, and the other resting on your knee.

2 Lift the weight up towards your chest and back down again. Repeat eight times, focusing on the back muscles, which are the ones doing the work.

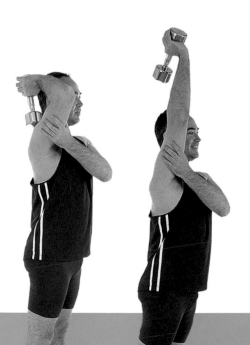

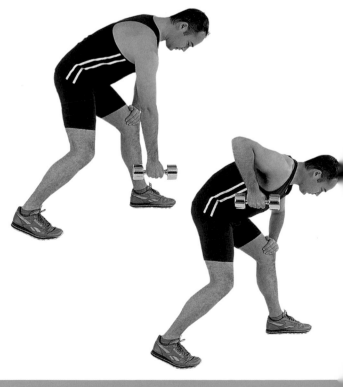

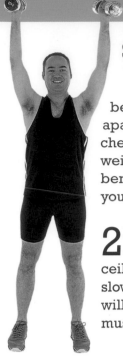

Shoulder press

1 Stand with your knees slightly bent, feet hip-width apart and ribcage and chest lifted. With a weight in each hand bend your arms to your shoulders.

2 Press the weights directly up to the ceiling and lower slowly. Eight repetitions will work your shoulder muscles (the deltoids).

Lie flat flies

1 Lie on your step bench with a weight in each hand. Extend your arms to the side but don't lock the elbows.

2 Bring the arms slowly towards each other to touch the dumbbells. Open your arms again.

3 Repeat eight times to strengthen the chest muscles (the pectorals).

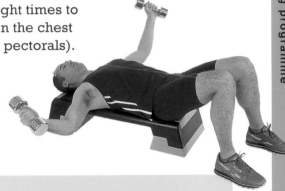

Technique Points

▶ The important thing for this workout is to discover which weight is your 'eight rep max'. Perform the exercises, either increasing or reducing weight so that eight repetitions is the most you can manage!

Muscle Strengthener: Ab weighted curls *repeat 20 times*

1 Lie on your back and hold a weight between your knees by squeezing with your inner thighs.

2 Now bring your legs towards yourself slightly and contract your abdominal muscles so that you lift your hips off the floor. Lift your upper body to meet your legs. Lower yourself with control.

3 Once you improve your strength you can perform this move with a smaller leg-swing at the beginning. Always keep a gap between your chin and chest.

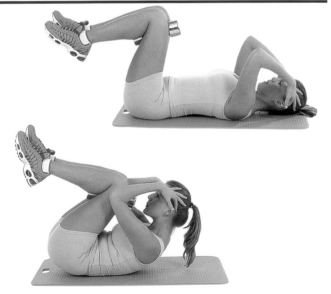

87

day 19

DON'T FORGET
▶ To warm up before (see pages 48–49)
▶ To cool down after (see pages 50–51)

Aerobic Exercise: Running 2 – *'Fartlek', or speed play running*

Fartlek is the Swedish word for speed play. The basic challenge is to incorporate several types of running in your session. If possible, do this session on grass. To start with, make the session last no longer than 20 minutes.

1 Run at a comfortable pace for five minutes then sprint until you reach the first person you see approaching you.

Bonus Burner

▶ Make the steady runs between components shorter (your recovery rate will improve as you get fitter), include more sprints, make the components last longer, or simply make the whole session last longer by doing more components. This is an excellent session for getting you out of your comfort zone.

2 Run at a comfortable pace for 30 seconds; then run 'knees to chest' for 30 seconds; run at a comfortable pace for another 30 seconds; then run sideways until you reach a landmark in the distance.

3 Run at a comfortable pace again, then race/walk until you reach a distant landmark.

4 After the first five minutes of steady running, include components such as sprinting, running sideways, long stride running, running 'vertically' emphasizing bringing your knees up to your chest, and race/walking emphasizing lateral hip movement.

5 Play with your speed and your steps. Make sure the final two or three minutes are of a steady nature.

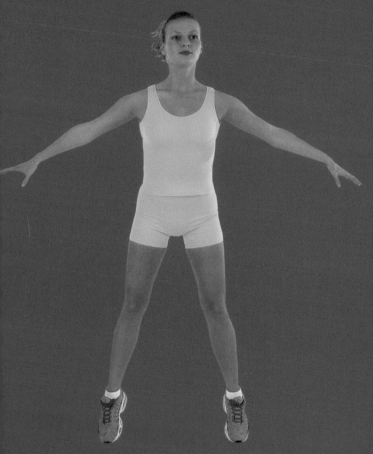

Technique Points

▶ As with all running sessions, maintain a good posture. This means your foot lands in a heel–toe sequence; it also means trying to keep your weight over your hips and not sagging.

▶ Stretch out rather than muscle strengthen for the end of this session. Do the stretches below, plus all the cooling down stretches (see pages 50–51).

Finishing Stretch:
Hip flexor

1 To stretch out the front of the hips, assume the position below and press the back hip forwards to feel the stretch.

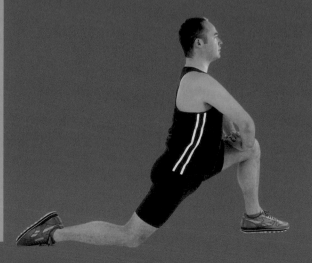

day 20

DON'T FORGET
► To warm up before (see pages 48–49)
► To cool down after (see pages 50–51)

Aerobic Exercise: Pyramid circuit with Swiss ball 2

Perform a continuous circuit of the following exercises with a Swiss ball, using the same pyramid principle as Days 8 and 11 (see pages 66–67 and 72–73). At each station perform 10 complete repetitions of the exercise. Between each level perform a 1-minute exercise 'break': jog for 1 minute while swinging the Swiss Ball over your head.

● **Station 1: Abdominal curls, lift and lowers**

1 Lie on your back and drape your legs over the ball, flexing the feet. Use your inner thigh muscles to hold the ball in place.

2 Now contract the abdominal muscles to bring the ball in towards your chest. Release back to the floor.

● **Station 2: Swiss ball side curl-ups**

1 Sit on the ball and gently walk your feet out so that the ball rolls underneath your lower back.

2 Place your hands behind your head. Raise your left knee towards your chest and bring your right elbow to meet it, performing a curl up. Repeat with your other knee.

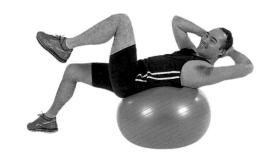

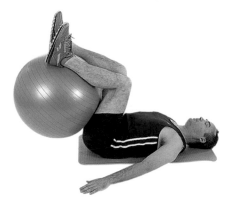

● **Station 3: Back arm and leg lift**

1 Drape yourself over the ball. Slowly lift your opposite arm and leg and hold, before releasing slowly down. This exercise will work the back and leg muscles. Repeat with the other arm and leg.

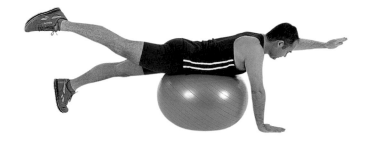

● Station 4: **Press-ups on ball**

1 Lie on top of the ball, face down, and take your weight on to your hands.

2 Slowly walk your hands out so that the ball rolls down towards your ankles. Use your knees and then your feet to control the ball.

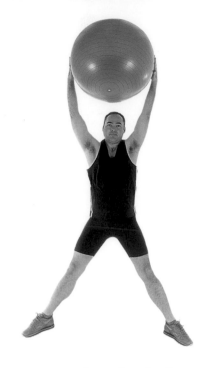

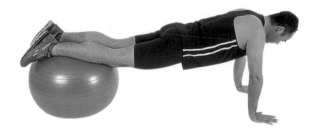

3 Bend and straighten your arms as before.

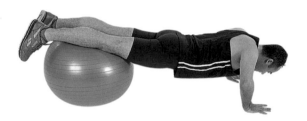

● Station 5: **Jumping jacks**

1 Jump with your arms up high holding on to the Swiss ball, landing with both feet wide apart. Bend the knees gently as you land. Repeat in rhythm.

● Station 6: **Ball balancing on knees**

1 Rest one knee on the ball first and then using your stomach muscles to help you keep straight, lift the second knee and try to balance momentarily with both knees on the ball. This is quite a feat so it will need practice!

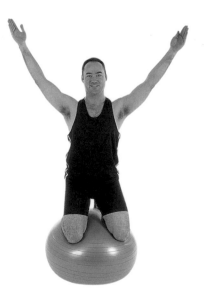

day 21

DON'T FORGET
► To warm up before (see pages 48–49)
► To cool down after (see pages 50–51)

Anaerobic Exercise: Mid-section weights workout

Today you are pushing the muscles hard, so as on Day 18 (pages 86–87), the workout is NOT about keeping going for 20 minutes. Use dumbbells that are heavy enough to challenge you after eight to ten repetitions (see Technique Points, page 87).

Side bends

1 Stand with your feet hip-width apart and your knees slightly bent. Pull in on your abdominals and lift your chest.

2 Grasp a weight in one hand and hold it by your side. Now let the weight tilt you over. Maintain this pose while you check that you are not arching your back or bending forward.

3 Now contract the oblique muscles (the sides of the abdominal area) to bring you back to the upright position. Do eight repetitions on each side to tone the sides of the stomach.

Lateral raises

1 Stand with your feet hip-width apart, knees slightly bent. Pull in on your abdominals and lift your chest. Holding a weight in each hand, and keeping your arms slightly bent and rounded, lift them out to the sides until they are parallel with the floor.

2 Hold this position momentarily and tip the end of the weights downwards and forwards slightly as if you are pouring from a jug. Then slowly lower your arms with control breathing freely throughout.

3 Do eight repetitions, focusing on the muscles that you are using at the sides of your torso.

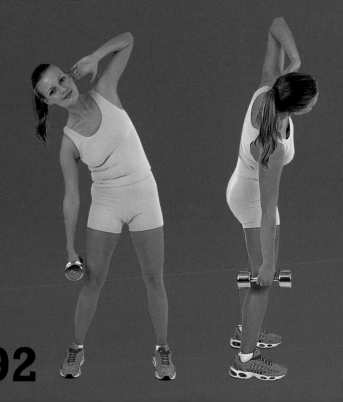

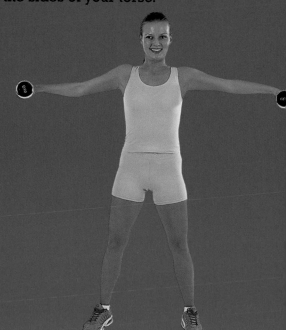

Cheating row

1 Step into a lunge position and lean forward, resting one hand on your thigh. Let the other arm, holding the weight, hang down to the floor.

2 Now pull up your arm, turning your body so that it faces to the side. Be sure to keep the supporting knee from twisting: the movement should be generated from the sides of the torso. Hold and release down.

3 Repeat eight times on each side. This is an excellent exercise for the back, shoulders and arms.

Muscle Strengthener: Ab weighted oblique curls

repeat 20 times

1 Lie on your back and hold a weight between your knees by squeezing it with your inner thighs.

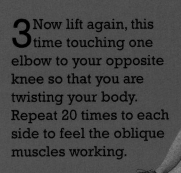

2 Now lift your head and shoulders with a hand on each ear. Lift, hold and release to the floor. Repeat 20 times. Always keep a gap between your chin and chest.

3 Now lift again, this time touching one elbow to your opposite knee so that you are twisting your body. Repeat 20 times to each side to feel the oblique muscles working.

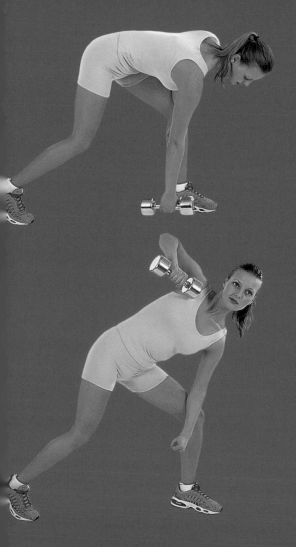

day 22

DON'T FORGET
► To warm up before (see pages 48–49)
► To cool down after (see pages 50–51)

Aerobic Exercise: Aerobic dance

This is another creative workout – now is your chance to practise all those funky aerobics moves. Aim to keep going non-stop for 20–25 minutes. If you run out of ideas jog on the spot while you think up some more!

Spotty dogs

1 Jump, throwing forward the arm and leg on the same side of your body, then swap to the other side as if you are doing an uncoordinated jerky walk!

Grapevines

1 Step to the side with your right foot, then step behind it with your left.

Jumping jacks

1 Jump with your arms out high and to the sides, landing with your feet wide apart. Bend the knees gently as you land. Repeat in rhythm.

2 Step to the side with your right foot again and bring the left foot over so your feet are together.

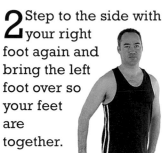

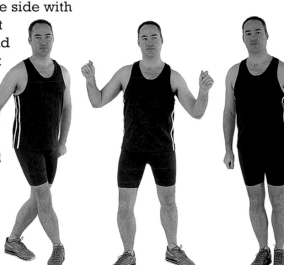

Bonus Burner

► Perform the moves above for four to five minutes then add in an up-and-down-stairs interval; if you can, sprint to the nearest tree. Then perform 20 burpees (see Day 3, page 57). Repeat the whole sequence four times.

Jump turns

1 Jump with a turn each time, to face each side of the room in turn.

Twister

1 Give your waist a good workout by jumping up and down, twisting your hips one way, then the other.

Lunge jumps

1 Assume the lunge position (see Day 13, page 76), and from here push upwards into a jump.

2 Land back down into the lunge, going through the feet and bending the knees so that there is no jarring on the legs. Change legs and repeat.

Recovery moves

1 These involve jogging on the spot, rope skipping on the spot (don't bother with the rope – just keep jumping), mini sprints up and down your living room and hopscotch.

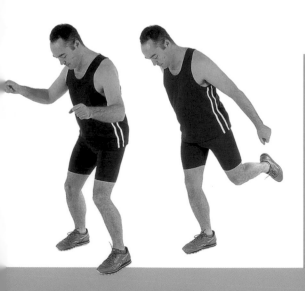

Muscle Strengthener:
Abductor toners

repeat 15 times on each leg

1 Lie on your side, propping yourself up on one elbow.

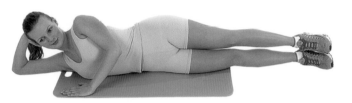

2 Make sure you keep your hips facing the side as you lift one leg high into the air and lower it again. If you are correctly positioned you will be able to lift the leg only up to a certain height. Lift the full range of movement and then lower with control.

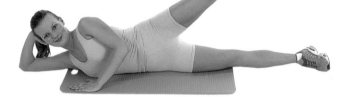

3 Perform 15 of these on each leg to tone the outer thighs.

Technique Points

▶ Keep your abdominals pulled in so that they support your torso at all times during this workout.

▶ When you jump make sure you land by rolling through the foot from toe to heel and then bending your knees.

day 23

DON'T FORGET
▶ To warm up before (see pages 48–49)
▶ To cool down after (see pages 50–51)

Aerobic Exercise: Pyramid circuit training 2

Perform a continuous circuit of the following exercises using the pyramid principle as used and explained first on Day 8 (see pages 66–67). The exercises involve anaerobic rather than aerobic work to really push up the heart rate. Muscle is the main performer here. At each station perform 10 complete repetitions of the exercise. Between each level perform a 1-minute exercise 'break': jog on the spot for 1 minute, raising your knees as high as you can lift them.

● **Station 1: Full press-ups** (see Day 15, page 81) Support yourself in the plank position with your hands and feet. Use your arms to raise and lower your chest.

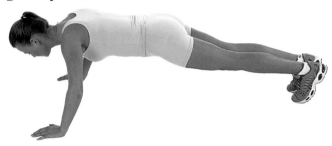

● **Station 2: Jumping jacks** (see Day 22, page 94) Jump with your arms straight out and land with your feet wide apart.

● **Station 3: Spotty dogs** (see Day 22, page 94) Jump, throwing forward your right leg and arm, then your left. Continue taking jerky steps.

● **Station 4: Lunge jumps** (see Day 13, page 76) Assume a lunge position but this time push upwards into a jump.

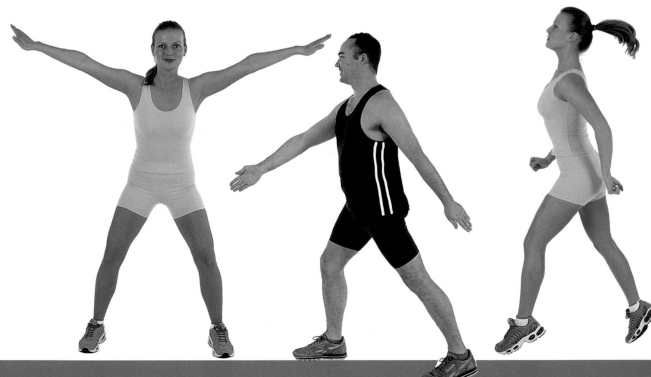

● **Station 5: Burpees** (see Day 3, page 57) Shoot your legs out behind you from a squat position then leap straight in the air with your arms outstretched. Try to get into a rhythm.

● **Station 6: Knee-to-chest jumps** (see Day 4, page 58, but without rebounder) Try to tuck your knees into your chest as you jump as high as possible. Bend your knees as you land.

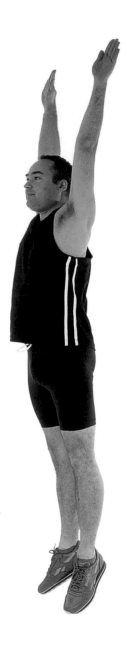

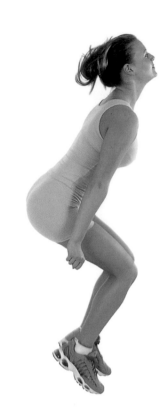

Technique Points

▶ Keep the jogging in the break as high as you can to really push yourself.

▶ Make sure each repetition of the ten you do on each level of the pyramid is executed as perfectly as the first.

day 24

DON'T FORGET
► To warm up before (see pages 48–49)
► To cool down after (see pages 50–51)

Anaerobic Exercise: Lower body weights

This is another workout with your 'eight rep max' (see Technique Points, page 87). If you have a barbell this will give an extra dimension to the moves. If you don't have one then simply use a pair of dumbbells.

Squats

1 Pick up and place the barbell across your shoulders. Position your feet hip-width apart and pull in on the abdominals for support.

Lunges

1 With the bar placed across your shoulders, step into a wide lunge position.

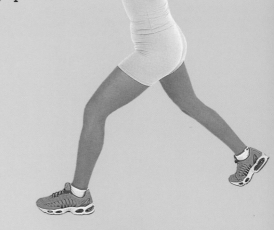

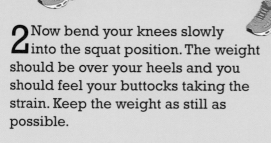

2 Now bend your knees slowly into the squat position. The weight should be over your heels and you should feel your buttocks taking the strain. Keep the weight as still as possible.

3 Press back up to standing. Repeat eight times.

2 Now lower your hips towards the floor by bending both legs equally. Press up to the start position. Repeat eight times.

Pliés

1 With the bar placed across your shoulders, step into a wide 'second position' (meaning that your feet are wider apart than the width of your hips), with your feet slightly turned out.

2 Slowly bend your knees with control, pressing them out exactly over the toes and feeling the muscles of the buttocks and backs of the legs working to maintain the position. Do not push your bottom out behind you (which would be a squat), but keep it between your hips.

3 Bend your knees until they are at right angles, then press up to the start position. Repeat eight times.

Muscle Strengthener:
Side leg lifts *repeat eight to ten times on each leg*

1 Stand one end of the barbell on the floor, and hold the other end for balance as you transfer your weight on to one leg.

2 Pull up in the abdominals and ribcage and lift the other leg out to the side as high as you can. Hold and then slowly lower. Straighten your arm for balance if necessary.

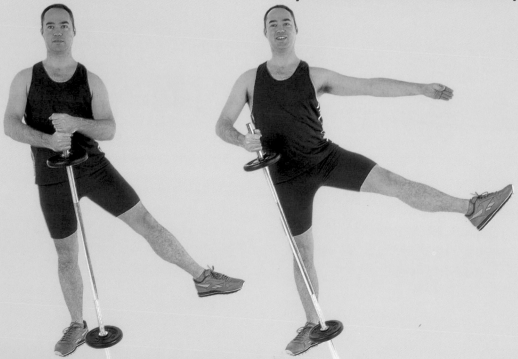

day 25

DON'T FORGET
► To warm up before (see pages 48–49)
► To cool down after (see pages 50–51)

Anaerobic Exercise: Plyometrics 2

Use the park, or your living room, for this workout. Warm up by walking briskly or jogging for five minutes, then try the following moves to vary your forward progress. In between each of the following moves jog on the spot to recover. This will take about 15 minutes.

Push off jumps

1 Crouch down low and steady yourself with your fingertips.

2 Push off with both legs and spring into the air. As you land bend your knees and slowly drop back into the starting position.

3 Try to do four lots of five jumps – but your legs may give up before that!

Burpees 2

1 Perform the basic burpees move (see Day 3, page 57): start in a low squat position, then shoot your legs out behind you.

2 Now jump the legs open into a straddle position, then bend your arms to do a press-up, tuck the legs back in and spring up to start the next repetition. Do 25 repetitions.

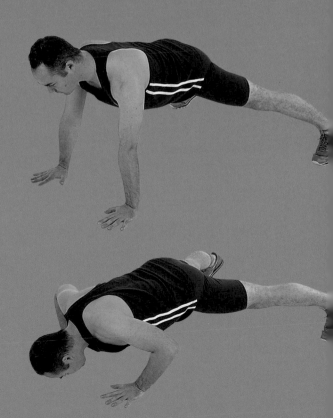

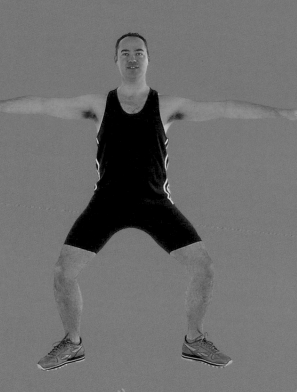

Technique Points

▶ It is important when doing any kind of jump that you check the alignment of your knees. As your knees bend, make sure that they are in line with your toes and not beyond them.

Muscle Strengthener: Jack-knife dorsal lifts

repeat 20 times

1 Assume the press-up position and hold. Now lift up your bottom and push with your arms and shoulders to form an inverted V-shape.

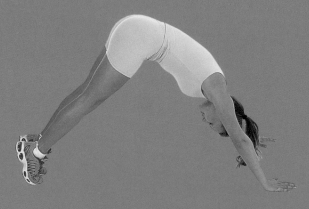

2 Lower yourself back to the press-up position and repeat. Use your stomach muscles to really lift the mid-section quickly.

Wide jumps

1 Stand with your legs apart and bend your knees. Raise your arms so they are parallel with the floor.

2 Spring off the floor and, while in the air, bring your legs together and your arms above your head. Land with your legs apart.

3 Perform 15 of these. Bend deeply as you land, so as to find the spring to keep the movement going.

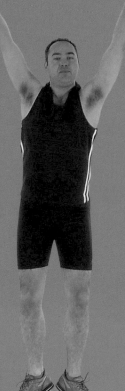

101

day 26

DON'T FORGET
▶ To warm up before (see pages 48–49)
▶ To cool down after (see pages 50–51)

Aerobic Exercise: Running 3 – *Triangle run*

Warm up first then find a triangular piece of land and repeat the steps below. Try to keep going for 20–30 minutes.

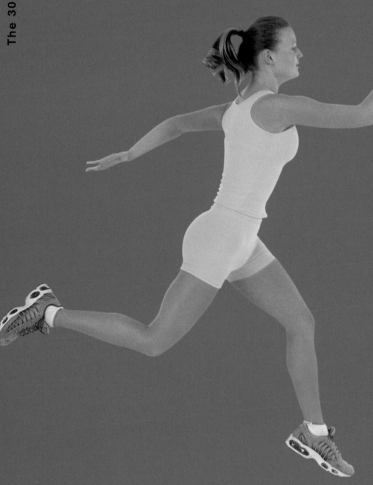

1 Run at a comfortable pace along the first side of the triangle, sprint along the second side, then run at a comfortable pace again along the third side to bring you back to the start. Then sprint on side one, run at a comfortable pace on side two, and sprint along side three.

2 Consider these two repetitions as one set, then jog on the spot for a short while and repeat a second set of two repetitions of this triangle.

3 Instead of sprinting, try bringing your knees to your chest in a vertical manner while running forward at the same time – this is tough! Or try running sideways along one segment of the triangle.

Bonus Burner

▶ Increase the repetitions in each set or increase the number of sets. Find a triangle with a hill in it. Sprinting up and down hills is fun!

▶ Reduce the amount of time between sets.

Technique Points

▶ Make sure you jog at a comfortable pace for five minutes at the end before finishing by stretching out (see pages 50–51).

▶ As with all running sessions maintain a good posture: this means your foot lands in a heel–toe sequence. It also means trying to keep your weight over your hips and not sagging.

Muscle Strengthener: Reverse press-up *repeat five times*

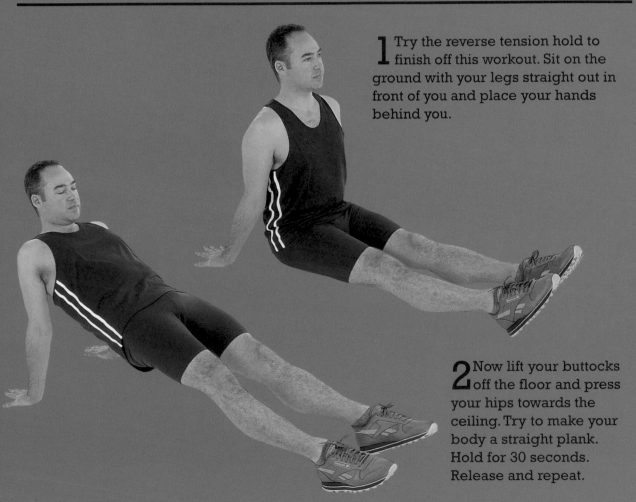

1 Try the reverse tension hold to finish off this workout. Sit on the ground with your legs straight out in front of you and place your hands behind you.

2 Now lift your buttocks off the floor and press your hips towards the ceiling. Try to make your body a straight plank. Hold for 30 seconds. Release and repeat.

103

day 27

DON'T FORGET
▶ To warm up before (see pages 48–49)
▶ To cool down after (see pages 50–51)

Aerobic Exercise: Step routine 2

This is a variation and expansion on the first step routine. Use the ideas from Day 2, page 55, and add the moves below to keep going for 30–40 minutes.

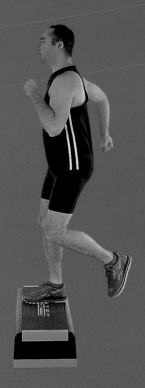
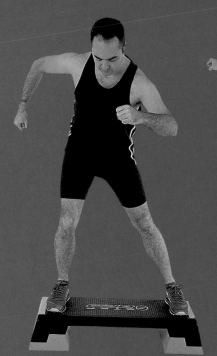
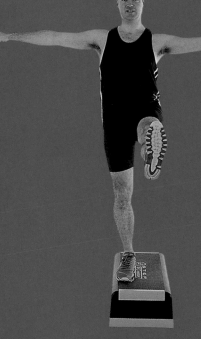

1 Step up and down for five minutes at a comfortable pace.

2 Increase the pace for another five minutes.

3 Now add some different steps: step wide on to the step and narrow as you step back down.

4 Step sideways on to the step and back down – add a kick on the top of your step.

Bonus Burner

▶ Carry dumbbells to add resistance.

▶ For some of the time jog on to the step bench rather than stepping on to it, but make sure you step back down.

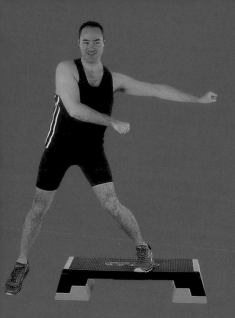

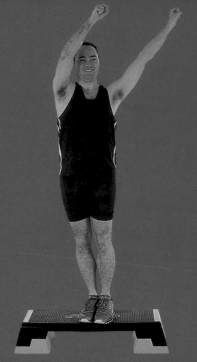

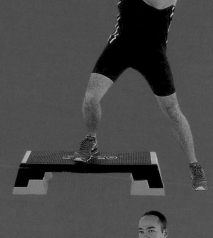

5 Step over the top of your step and down the other side; when you master this, jump this move. Wave your arms around as you move.

6 Lunge off one side and lunge jump to the other side (see Day 13, page 77).

Muscle Strengthener:
Step press-ups *repeat 15 times*

1 Now you are ready to try an advanced form of press-up. Position your feet on the step and your hands on the floor to perform 15 press-ups.

2 Rest and then attempt the same number with your hands on the bench in a narrow position. As you bend your arms, your elbows must be tucked right into the ribcage (not out at right angles as for a normal press-up). In this way you are focusing on the tricep muscles at the back of the arms.

Technique Points

▶ Keep the full foot on the step. Keep your knees bent slightly when on top of the step and keep your chest lifted.

▶ Try and keep the step action to a clear count of four in your head, i.e. up one, two; down three, four.

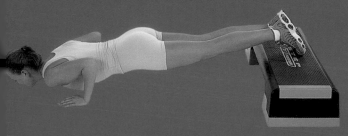

105

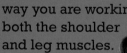
day 28

DON'T FORGET
► To warm up before (see pages 48–49)
► To cool down after (see pages 50–51)

Anaerobic Exercise: Combination weights

For this workout you will need to use lighter weights than your 'eight rep max' (see (see Technique Points, page 87). Each of these moves is a combination of two exercises so that you are doing twice the work in one move. Attempt each of these moves 10–15 times. Rest for 30 seconds between each move. Repeat whole circuit two or three times.

Shoulder shack

1 Hold a dumbbell in each hand and rest your hands on your shoulders.

2 Perform a squat move (see Day 24, page 98) and as you press upwards lift one leg up as high as you can while pressing the dumbbells towards the ceiling.

3 Return to the start position and repeat with the other leg. In this way you are working both the shoulder and leg muscles.

Slalom

1 Holding slightly lighter weights, use the squat position to jump and land.

2 As you jump, press your hips out to one side and then the other as if you are skiing down a fast snowy slope! Use your arms to push behind you as if you were holding ski poles.

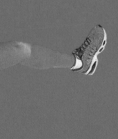

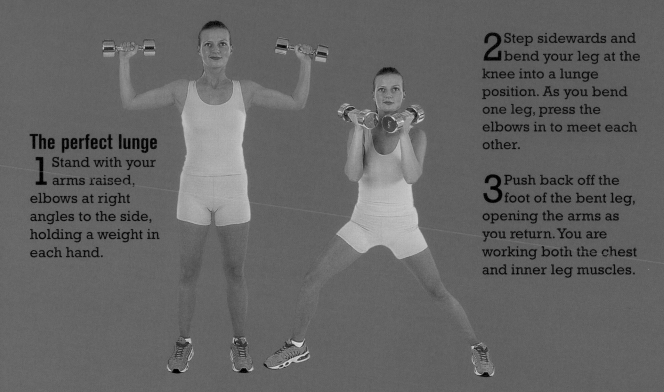

The perfect lunge

1 Stand with your arms raised, elbows at right angles to the side, holding a weight in each hand.

2 Step sidewards and bend your leg at the knee into a lunge position. As you bend one leg, press the elbows in to meet each other.

3 Push back off the foot of the bent leg, opening the arms as you return. You are working both the chest and inner leg muscles.

Muscle Strengthener:
One leg tri *repeat ten times on each leg*

1 Stand and take the weight off one leg but keep those toes on the floor for balance. Holding weights in each hand, lift the elbows up and back behind you for the start position.

2 Slowly squat and press the arms straight as you lower yourself. Check the alignment of your knee, ensuring it goes directly over the toe, as you lower. Use that leg to press yourself to the start position, slowly bending the arms again.

3 Perform ten on one leg and then ten on the other. This works both the arm and leg muscles.

Technique Points

▶ Keep your breathing regular throughout these exercises and keep the abdominals tight to support the torso at all times. Focus equally on both the contraction (the beginning) and release phase of the movements.

day 29

DON'T FORGET
▶ To warm up before (see pages 48–49)
▶ To cool down after (see pages 50–51)

Aerobic Exercise: Football circuit 2

This workout mimics football activities for training/fitness purposes. Start by placing a line of perhaps six markers directly behind one another, about 10 metres (10 yards) apart, or use trees in a park and keep moving for about 30 minutes.

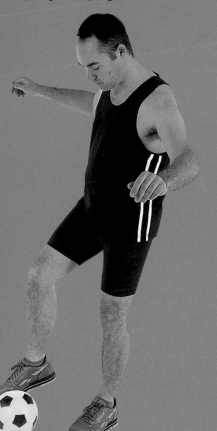

1 Sprint to the first marker, touch the ground, turn and sprint back to the start.

2 Then sprint to the second and back in the same way. Continue for 25 minutes, taking in all the markers and adding in the variations listed.

Variations:

There are some interesting variations you can try.

▶ Instead of touching the ground as you turn, leap up in the air as if to head a ball. This is tiring!

▶ Try running as fast as you can to each marker while controlling a ball.

▶ Try sprinting to each marker, jumping in the air twice then jogging back to the start while balancing the ball on your head!

Bonus Burner

▶ Increase the number of markers and variations you do. Aim, eventually, to have as short a recovery time as possible between sets – rapid recovery in football matches is vital for good play.

▶ Pretend you are taking a free kick towards one of the six markers. Hone your skill by trying to land the ball as close as possible to each marker you aim at. Sprint to the marker, then kick the ball back as close to the start as you can get it. Do a set and time yourself.

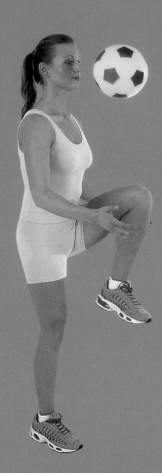

Muscle Strengthener:
Football skills

Bouncing ball off knees - repeat 100 times

1 Try to bounce the ball off your knees so that it does not fall to the ground. This exercise is good for coordination. Try and alternate the legs that you are using.

2 Keep your stomach pulled up, so that you can lift your legs nice and high and keep breathing as you concentrate.

3 Aim to keep the ball bouncing for 100 bounces. If you drop the ball, start again!

Ab ball extension - repeat 20 times

1 Sit down with the football between your heels and your hands behind to support you.

2 Now lean back and straighten your legs briefly then recoil to the start position.

3 Repeat, sending your feet slightly off to one side then the other. Do 20 repetitions to feel the stomach really working.

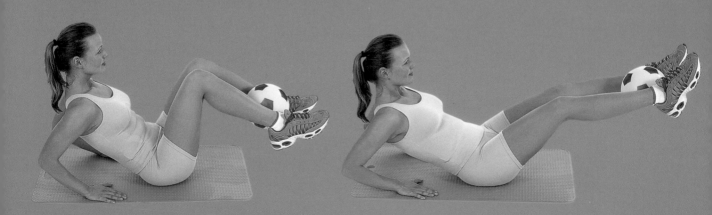

day 30

DON'T FORGET
▶ To warm up before (see pages 48–49)
▶ To cool down after (see pages 50–51)

Aerobic Exercise: Running 4 - *Interval training*

After a good warm-up perform sprints of various intervals in a park or around a running track for up to 30 minutes.

1 Try to sprint for 30 seconds then jog for 30 seconds. Repeat this three times. Jog for one minute then repeat the whole lot twice more.

2 Alternatively, sprint for 30 seconds, jog for 30 seconds, sprint for 40 seconds, jog for 40 seconds and continue like this adding ten seconds each time, to a maximum of 90 seconds.

3 Instead of time segments use distance segments – sprint 100 metres (100 yards), jog 100 metres (100 yards) and so on. To increase your endurance, run at about 80 per cent effort for longer segments such as one or even two minutes.

Bonus Burner

▶ Increase the number of sets you run!

▶ Increase the number of repetitions in each set, or decrease the amount of jogging recovery between repetitions. Increase the intensity of the endurance components.

▶ An alternative muscle-building exercise is to kick up to a handstand against the wall, if you can, and hold it for one minute. Repeat.

Technique Points

▶ As with all running sessions maintain a good posture: this means your foot lands in a heel–toe sequence. It also means trying to keep your weight over your hips and not sagging.

Muscle Strengthener: Isometric circular press

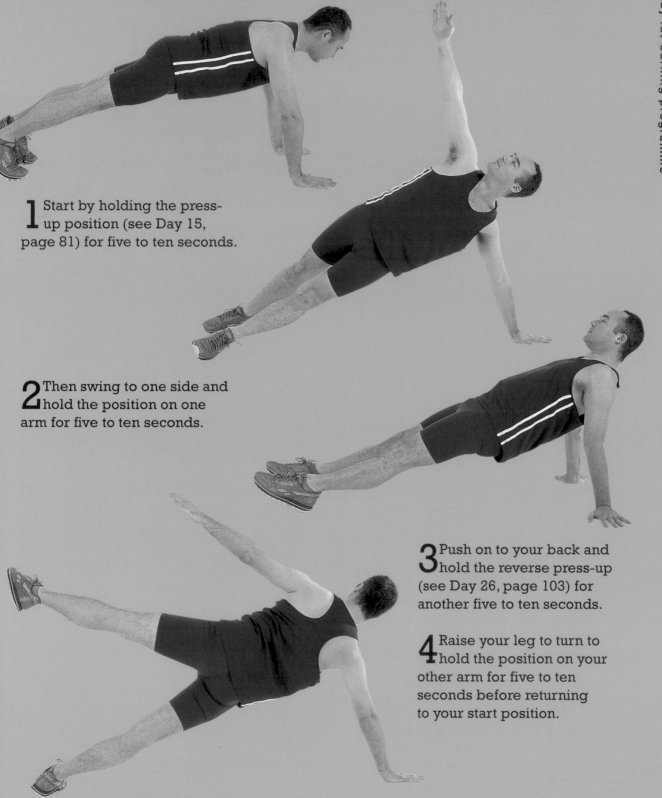

1 Start by holding the press-up position (see Day 15, page 81) for five to ten seconds.

2 Then swing to one side and hold the position on one arm for five to ten seconds.

3 Push on to your back and hold the reverse press-up (see Day 26, page 103) for another five to ten seconds.

4 Raise your leg to turn to hold the position on your other arm for five to ten seconds before returning to your start position.

Maintaining your new figure

Congratulations! By now you should have completed the 30-day programme – or at least finished reading it! Your challenge now is to maintain your new-found energy and figure.

You may find, now that you have made the initial effort, that you don't need to exercise every single day and therefore you can start to pick and choose areas of the programme to keep your fitness and figure at a constant level.

If you are happy to exercise on three days a week and you find that this keeps your fat levels where you want them, then choose three different routines from the programme, to focus on each week.

If you want to 'spot tone' problem areas, then use the suggestions opposite to target those areas in the best way possible.

Then, once a year, try to go right through the whole 30-day programme again for one month just to get your fitness levels right up again. This way you can make the programme work for you and keep it working for you for many years to come!

Pick and choose

If you are feeling a bit off-form, need to try to blitz the fat-burning or have less time than usual, then pick one of these three alternatives below.

The easier week – If you are feeling a little under the weather and want to give yourself an easier routine for a week or two then try this combination of workouts.
Week 1:   Days 1, 3, 5, plus muscle strengtheners from Days 1, 2 and 4
Week 2:   Days 4, 9, 11, plus muscle strengtheners from Days 1, 2 and 4

Mega-cardiovascular – Lost your way a little and piled on a few pounds? Try this combination for four days a week for three weeks, to pull you back on track.
Week 1:   Days 1, 2, 13, 29
Week 2:   Days 15, 7, 10, 27
Week 3:   Days 19, 25, 26, 30

Short-of-time week – Use the pyramid on Days 8 and 11 but cut down the number of stations if you're really short of time. Or use the circuit session on Day 6 and cut the time on each station to one minute and repeat the circuit just twice.

Spot-toning problem areas

As we have already seen (page 19) you cannot choose the area of your body from which you want to burn fat. However, you can spot-tone specific muscles.

Target your lower body – Want to focus on your legs and bottom a little more? Try this combination of workouts for two weeks.

Week 1: Muscle strengtheners from Days 4, 6, 7, 10, 11, 12
Week 2: Muscle strengtheners from Days 15, 16, 19, 23, 30

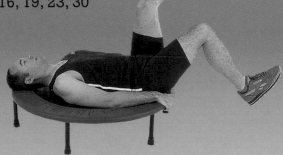

Target your upper body – Try this combination of workouts for two weeks if you want to focus on your upper body.

Week 1: Muscle strengtheners from Days 3, 5, 6, 8, 9
Week 2: Muscle strengtheners from Days 11, 14, 17, 18, 21

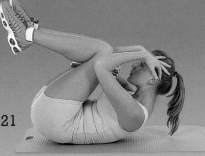

Target your middle – Tone up the stomach and back with these aerobic and muscle-strengthening exercises.

Week 1: Days 3, 5, plus muscle strengtheners from Days 2, 4, 6, 14, 15, 16
Week 2: Days 8, 18, plus muscle strengtheners from Days 17, 18, 21, 25, 26, 29, 30

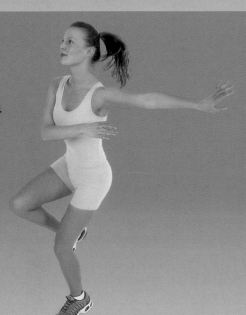

114

5 Burning fat anywhere

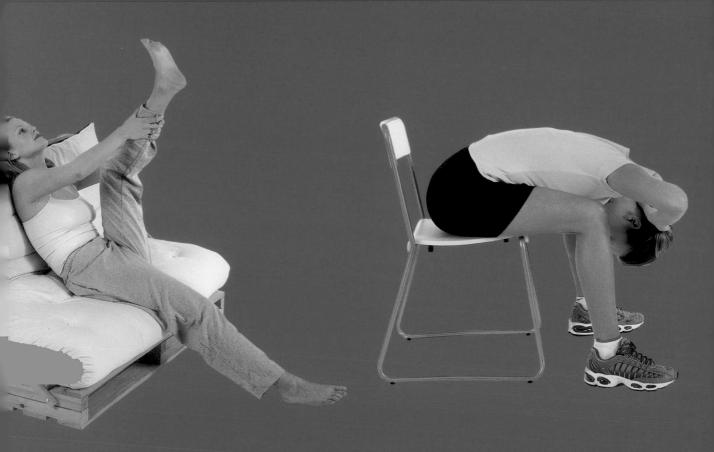

Get more exercise into your life

The knowledge we gain in life is forever changing and evolving. As science progresses we discover more about our body's systems and issues such as obesity and weight loss.

Certain studies suggest that some people seem to be able to eat more and put on less weight than others. Other studies suggest that these people are simply more active without realizing it. When you tap your foot or pace up and down the room during a phone call, for example, you are using up calories. These actions may be the reason behind some people's seemingly effortless weight control. On the other hand, some people have a smaller appetite – eating only until they are no longer hungry – not until they are full. Certainly, appetite is a key area that scientists are looking at in a bid to understand weight gain.

Until scientists have the definitive answer, or produce a pill that simply dissolves fat as we make it – exercising is the key to maintaining a healthy weight. Exercise will help to keep the body healthy and in good working order.

Aside from the periods you have set aside for working out, the following pages provide some suggestions for getting more exercise or action into your everyday life. You may choose not to follow these ideas, but keeping them in mind will increase your exercise options.

Active appraisal

Start by assessing exactly how many journeys you make that are less than a mile, or a couple of kilometres. How often do you drive these short journeys? Well why not walk them instead? It's more environmentally friendly, it will get you out and about in your local neighbourhood and it will burn you some extra calories. It may take a little time – plan to factor in an extra ten minutes of walking time here and there – but you will be repaid tenfold in terms of relaxation and health.

Next, factor into your day some little exercise extras. Remember, the people who stay naturally slim probably do a lot more exercise than you realize.

Escalate your activity

Whenever you go out and about – take the most active route possible. Watch kids. They are great at getting the most out of every landscape and making it into a playground. If there is something they can climb over they will! If there is something they can slide under they will! So:
▶ Take the stairs instead of the lift.
▶ If there is an escalator, keep walking as it carries you up.
▶ Sprint for the bus and cycle to work if you can.

Make a stretch start

Start your day with a few stretches. They don't need to be anything fancy or complicated but they will wake you up and get you going in the morning.

Add any other stretches you enjoy or have come across – or do something completely different! But starting your day with movement will get both your body and mind ready for the day – and you will have burned some calories!

Morning full stretch

1 Sit up with your legs stretched out together in front of you. Reach up to the sky with your arms clasped above your head.

2 Flex and extend your feet – contracting the calves will get the blood flowing, particularly through the veins, on the way back up to the heart.

Morning wide-legged stretch

1 Sit up with your legs apart and stretched out in front of you.

2 Lean forward, stretching your arms in front of you as far as you can reach.

Morning cross-legged stretch

1 Sit on the bed with your legs in front of you. Cross one leg over the other and twist your top half around to look over one shoulder to wake up your torso.

2 Cross the other leg over the top and twist round to the other side.

Morning side stretch

1 Sit cross-legged on the bed. Extend one arm above your head and bend over to the opposite side.

2 Now repeat with the other arm and tip to the other side.

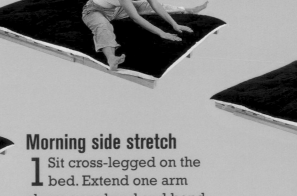

TV active

Many of us like to watch television at the end of a hard day, and why not? If it helps relax your mind and helps you unwind then it's all to the good. Use it wisely, however. You don't need to watch those car adverts all the time, do you? So why not use those breaks to stretch?

Full body stretch

1 Lie back on your couch and reach your arms up to the ceiling. Arch your back, push your bottom into the cushions, straighten your legs and get a really great stretch along the whole front of your body.

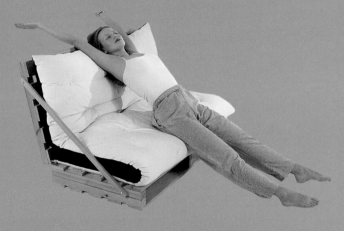

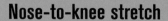

Leg stretch

1 Sit back in the couch, lift one leg up towards your hands and gently pull the leg towards you, so that you stretch out the back of the leg. Repeat with the other leg.

Nose-to-knee stretch

1 Lie on your back on the couch and lift one leg in the air. Now curl up your head and shoulders and try and touch your nose to your knee. Repeat on each leg until your TV programme restarts.

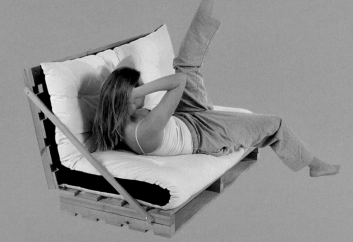

End of day deeds

Why not use the end of the day to tack on a few exercises before you go to bed? Although the end of the day is not the best time to start an intense exercise session as it will keep you awake, try doing a few of the muscle builders described in the 30-day programme or perform a few gentle stretches.

Leg stretch with towel

1 Lie flat on the bed with one leg raised and loop a towel around your foot. Gently pull the towel towards you. You will feel the back of the leg stretching.

2 Hold and repeat on the other leg. This stretches the hamstring muscle and relieves the tension in the back of the legs and calves, and can help prevent cramp at night.

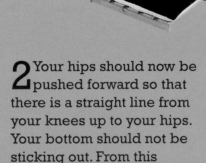

Three-quarter press-ups

1 Get on to all fours on the bed. Walk your hands out one step in front of you. Keep your knees where they are and swing your weight forward over your arms.

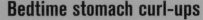

2 Your hips should now be pushed forward so that there is a straight line from your knees up to your hips. Your bottom should not be sticking out. From this 'three-quarter' position you can now perform press-ups by lowering and raising your arms.

3 As you push back with your arms, push right off and clap your hands before landing. Repeat 8–15 times.

Bedtime stomach curl-ups

1 Lie back on your bed and perform 50 curl-ups (see Day 2, page 55, but keep your feet on the mattress). The softness of the mattress helps you to really curl up high and strong. Use this time to work on your technique.

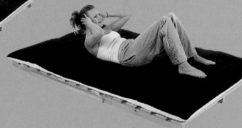

Deep breathing

1 Lie flat on the bed and breathe deeply. Deep breathing is good for the circulation and for winding the body down in preparation for rest.

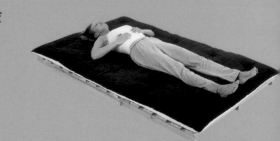

Exercising at work

Work is one of the hardest places in which to exercise – unless of course you're a fitness instructor! For a start, the workplace is not set up for you to work out and secondly there is always the next deadline to distract you from any thoughts of exercise.

Remember, however, that taking proper breaks will improve your performance, not detract from it. Moving around will get the blood flowing and allow oxygen to circulate freely, providing mental as well as physical inspiration!

If possible, set an alarm in your PC notebook or program your computer to remind you to move around every 30 minutes, and try stick to this reminder. If you can keep the body mobile throughout the day you will not only burn extra calories and avoid stiffness but also help yourself avoid varicose veins and the risk of deep vein thrombosis.

Finally, at the end of the day take a brisk walk homewards. If you have to use public transport then get off a stop earlier than you usually do to give yourself a longer walk than normal.

Office workout

Try the following exercises, which can be done at your work station, to keep moving onwards and upwards at work.

Body stretch

1 Relax your back and get the blood flowing to your head by leaning your full upper body over your legs. Let your head hang down and relax your arms. Breathe in and out slowly several times.

2 Finally, place your hands on your head and press your head in towards your knees to stretch out your neck. You can do this under your desk or away from it.

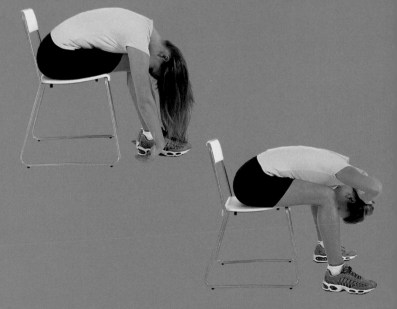

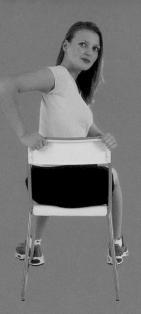

Body twist

1 Turn around on your chair until you can grip the back of it with both hands – if you can't do this straight away practise every day until you can.

2 Hold the position and twist a little farther. Repeat on the other side. This will help keep the blood flowing and aid flexibility in your torso.

Warm-up

1 If you sit for a long time you can become quite cold – this is a sure sign that you need to get active. Stand up, bend your knees and run on your toes as fast as you can.

2 By lifting your heels you can lift your knees up and run fast like a cartoon character! You will feel the work happening in the thighs and this will get the body heat and your breathing going.

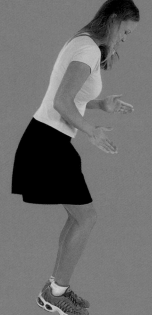

Knee lift

1 Get those legs moving and tone the thighs as you work! While you are sitting, lift one leg straight up so that the top of your toe touches the desk. Push as hard as you can against the underside of the desk.

2 Repeat with the other leg. Keep breathing (or even talking) while you do 20 of these on each leg.

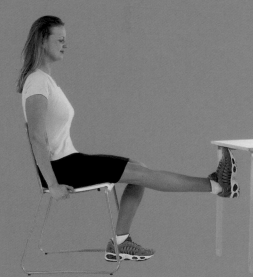

121

Ideas for the holiday season

When the holiday season looms, try not to let your new regime of exercise go out the window. Holidays are a time when one tends to overindulge and not feel like doing the old routine. That's fair enough but if you can keep some kind of exercise routine ticking over, you won't lose your fitness and it'll be easier to get back into it when the time comes.

Festive holidays

During festive holidays there are always lots of parties and social gatherings, taking up time and energy, so you may need to get your fitness routine down to a minimum.

Try performing some of the workouts that are based more indoors such as the step routine (see Days 2, page 54 and 27, page 104) and the shadow boxing (see Days 3, page 56 and 14, page 78) or the Pyramids (see Days 8, page 66 and 23, page 96). These routines require a minimum of equipment and you can also cut the routine in half if you are really short of time. With the Pyramid particularly, if you have time for only a 15-minute workout then shave off one block of the pyramid, giving you a short, yet still 'complete' workout.

If you know you have a big event to attend and you will be drinking and eating a lot then make sure you fit in a workout beforehand. This will increase your calorie needs and your metabolism will be raised – just what you need to deal with the extra intake. Not only

this, but if you do some exercise it will fire you up and keep your energy levels high for the party!

On your return from the party, drink plenty of water to help your system if you have overindulged. If you have eaten too much and are feeling bloated and nauseous, hit the floor and do 20–30 press-ups! Start using up some of that food you just ate and give your stomach some room!

Traditional gifts for many festive holidays are usually laden with chocolate – so keep exercising if you don't want to gain extra pounds. Chocolate is full of sugar which can give you quite dramatic energy highs and lows. Do lots of cardiovascular (CV) work to keep the body on a level. Use the routines on Day 1 (page 52) and Days 7 (page 64), 9 (page 68), 26 (page 102) and 30 (page 110), which involve walking and running. Change your route a bit when you run and discover something new in your area.

Summer holidays

Going away for a summer break is the perfect opportunity to work out with a difference. A varied routine will keep you from becoming bored and a change of scenery is as good as anything.

Be sure to pack your skipping rope so you can do the routine on Day 15 (page 80) and do the running routines on Days 7 (page 64), 9 (page 68), 26 (page 102) and 30 (page 110). They will offer you the chance to explore your new surroundings.

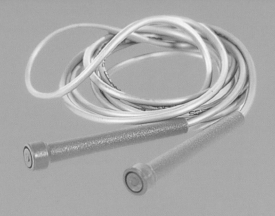

Swimming is another great CV exercise, so why not try the workout given below?

Aerobic Exercise: Swimming

Too often, people swim along in a complete comfort zone. The challenge here is to swim for 20 minutes out of your comfort zone.

1 Try swimming one length fast, one length slow. You could vary the workout by changing strokes every other length.

Bonus burner

▶ After a fast length, rest until partially recovered then swim another fast length.

▶ Build up to two lengths fast, one recovery.

▶ To add resistance, use buoyancy belts.

Muscle Strengthener: Leg lifts *repeat 20 times on each leg*

1 Now that you are nice and warm in the water, stand there with one hand on the side to balance you.

2 Lift one straight leg up until the foot comes out of the water and then lower it.

3 Repeat this 20 times on each leg. Lifting the leg in water is like lifting it with heavy weights on – so you'll really tone the thigh muscles.

Technique Points

▶ Wear goggles, which allow you to get your face underwater and thus give better stroke mechanics. Go on, get your hair wet!

▶ The fitter you are, the quicker your recovery heart rate will be. Check this in the pool (see page 29) while resting after a fast length.

123

Active weekend

While you are trying to keep your fitness programme regular, there are times when all your best-laid plans can go amiss. Maybe you have been ill or so inundated with work that your schedule has been hijacked. Well don't despair – remember that you can always get back on track if you restart your programme the following week. In the meantime, however, why not give yourself an active weekend to blow away the stress of the working week?

Walking

As well as the fitness walking programme included on Day 1, page 52, you can also try a more relaxed approach. Choose an area in your neighbourhood that you don't know so well and go and explore. Set yourself half an hour to walk about and have a really good look around you. Then you can turn around at 30 minutes and work your way back again.

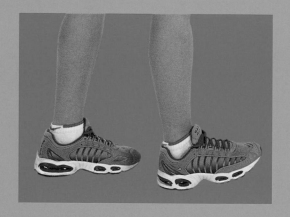

If you can, why not find a nearby hill, mountain or forest to hike across? Challenge yourself and try and walk or hike, with the aid of a big stick, as fast as you can. Even if you are confined to built-up areas you can still hike up the hills and steps in your local area.

▶ Hiking
▶ Roller-blading
▶ Rowing
▶ Windsurfing
▶ Diving
▶ Skateboarding
▶ Dry skiing

Active pursuits

There are many other active pursuits that you can try for a weekend. Most of the following can be done – or even attempted in a weekend – so why not try something new?

Domestic pursuits

If, however, you are confined to looking after your kids (or other people's!) for the weekend, then try taking them to the park where you can perform this workout.

Garden workout

This is a great workout to do in the privacy of your back garden making use of whatever children's play equipment you have. Jog around the garden for 10 minutes first to warm up.

Be sure to carefully check that the children's play equipment can take your full weight before carrying out these exercises.

1 If you have a climbing frame use it to do some hanging work. Hang off the bar and try to perform as many pull-ups as you can. This is a tough exercise and if you cannot manage to pull yourself up initially then jump up to the up position and slowly lower yourself down to the hang position. This will build up your strength.

2 Hang off the bar and lift your legs and feet up at right angles to your body. Do this ten times.

3 If there are some hanging handles hold on to them and see if you can turn yourself upside down!

4 If you have a large enough swing – sit on it and then, holding on to the chains with both hands, lift your bottom off the seat and lower it back down again. Repeat this ten times.

5 If you have a slide, place your hands at the bottom of the slide, adopt the press-up position and perform 20 press-ups.

6 Stand astride the bottom of the slide. Jump with both feet on to the slide and back down on to the floor again. Repeat ten times.

7 Now push the kids on the swings as hard as you can.

Muscle Strengthener: Leg lifts *repeat ten times on each leg*

1 Finally, use any other piece of equipment you can find, or even a chair from inside, that you can lift one leg upon.

2 Rest one heel on the chair then lift and lower that leg ten times. On the final rest, lean forward over that leg so that you stretch the hamstring.

3 Repeat with the other leg.

125

Index

Acknowledgements

Special thanks to **Physical Company**
(telephone: 01628 520208) for the supply
of equipment

Editor: Abi Rowsell

Executive Art Editor: Leigh Jones
Designer: Tony Truscott

Photographer: Peter Pugh-Cook
Models: Ildiko Vesei and Keith Brazil
Stylist: Aruna Mathur

Production Controller: Viv Cracknell